CHARLES B. INLANDER is president of the People's Medical Society. As chief executive officer since its founding in early 1983, Mr. Inlander has guided the People's Medical Society to its status as the largest non-profit consumer health advocacy organization in the country. He is the co-author of numerous books, including *Take This Book to the Hospital with You* and *Medicine on Trial*.

Mr. Inlander also serves as a lecturer at the Yale University School of Medicine and is a member of the board of directors of the Civil Justice Foundation and the National League for Health Care. He is on the editorial board of, and writes a column for, *Nursing Economics* magazine. His articles have also been printed in such publications as *The New York Times*, and he has appeared on numerous radio and television programs.

JIM PUNKRE is a freelance writer who has written about health, fitness, and nutrition for over twenty years.

An entrepreneur, he has worked in the fields of advertising, marketing, fund-raising, editing, art and design, and music. He is the creator of "Sound Medicine"—an audiocassette program of guided imagery and sound vibrations designed to relieve stress, lower blood pressure, and induce deep relaxation.

Mr. Punkre is currently the president of Brainstorms—a Newport Beach, California, corporation that provides creative services to firms specializing in direct marketing.

≡People's Medical Society.

HEALTHY BODY
▪ BOOK ▪

Test Yourself for
Maximum Health

CHARLES B. INLANDER
and JIM PUNKRE

Penguin Books

PENGUIN BOOKS
Published by the Penguin Group
Viking Penguin, a division of Penguin Books USA Inc.,
375 Hudson Street, New York, New York 10014, U.S.A.
Penguin Books Ltd, 27 Wrights Lane, London W8 5TZ, England
Penguin Books Australia Ltd, Ringwood, Victoria, Australia
Penguin Books Canada Ltd, 2801 John Street, Markham, Ontario, Canada L3R 1B4
Penguin Books (N.Z.) Ltd, 182-190 Wairau Road, Auckland 10, New Zealand

Penguin Books Ltd, Registered Offices:
Harmondsworth, Middlesex, England

First published in Penguin Books 1991

10 9 8 7 6 5 4 3 2 1

A NOTE TO THE READER:
The ideas, procedures, and suggestions contained in this book are not intended
as a substitute for consulting with your physician. All matters regarding your
health require medical supervision.

LIBRARY OF CONGRESS CATALOGING IN PUBLICATION DATA
Inlander, Charles B.
People's Medical Society healthy body book : test yourself for
maximum health / Charles B. Inlander and Jim Punkre.
  p.   cm.
ISBN 0 14 01.5286 5
  1. Health—Miscellanea.   2. Self-care, Health—Miscellanea.
3. Consumer education.   I. Punkre, Jim.   II. People's Medical
Society (U.S.)   III. Title.
RA776.5.I55   1991
613—dc20   90–21468

Printed in the United States of America

Set in Century expanded
Text design by Beth Tondreau Design / Mary A. Wirth

CONTENTS

INTRODUCTION ▪ **ix**

1 ▪ WHO AM I? ▪ **1**
- How to Tell If You're Past Your Prime ▪ 2
- Are You a Thrillaholic? ▪ 11
- Intelligence Quiz: Are You Smart? ▪ 13
- The Love and Understanding Quiz ▪ 15
- Stress Rating Scale ▪ 28

2 ▪ YOU ARE WHAT YOU EAT! ▪ **31**
- How's Your Diet? ▪ 32
- Fast-Food Quiz ▪ 42
- Test Your Overall Nutrition Knowledge ▪ 49
- Are You Up on Your Facts About Fat? ▪ 53
- Are You at Risk of Obesity? ▪ 57
- Test Yourself: Vitamins ▪ 58

■ Do You Know Where the Sodium Is in Your Diet?   ■ 62
■ How Low Do You Go? Do You Know?   ■ 64
■ Testing Your Sodium Savvy   ■ 65

3 ■ CHECK YOURSELF OUT   ■ 71

■ Test Your Health IQ   ■ 72
■ How Fit Are You?   ■ 75
■ A Quick Test for Macular Disease, Thief of Central
Vision   ■ 78
■ Glaucoma: Are You at Risk?   ■ 79
■ How's Your Hearing?   ■ 80
■ Do Your Height and Weight See Eye to Eye?   ■ 82
■ How to Determine Your Target Heart Rate   ■ 85
■ How to Do Breast Self-Examination   ■ 87
■ Health IQ Quiz: Osteoporosis   ■ 90
■ A Self-Exam for Testicular Cancer   ■ 91
■ Vasectomy Myths: How Many Have You Fallen
For?   ■ 93
■ The Rockport Fitness Walking Test   ■ 96

4 ■ HOW'S YOUR CHILD?   ■ 108

■ What's Your Parenting Quotient?   ■ 109
■ How Balanced Is Your Child's Diet?   ■ 117
■ Is Your Child Allergic?   ■ 121
■ Is Your Baby's Hearing Normal?   ■ 127
■ Simple Do-It-Yourself Scoliosis Check   ■ 130
■ How Fit Are Your Kids?   ■ 132
■ Is Your Playground Safe?   ■ 136
■ How to Choose the Right Pediatrician   ■ 141
■ Parents' Rights: Do You Know Where You Stand?   ■ 145

5 ■ ARE YOU AN EMPOWERED
MEDICAL CONSUMER?   ■ 150

■ Your Medical Rights: Do You Really Know Them?   ■ 151
■ Where Are the Hazards in Modern Medicine? Do
You Know Enough to Avoid Them?   ■ 156

■ A Test About Unnecessary Testing ■ 159
■ Does Your Doctor Treat You with the Respect You
Deserve? ■ 164
■ Do You Know Which Medical Specialist Does
What—and Where? ■ 167
■ Do You Know Your Hospital Rights? ■ 171
■ Does Your Hospital Bill Pass This Test? ■ 177
■ Can You Read Your Medical Chart? ■ 181
■ Can You Read Your Prescription Form? ■ 184
■ Insurance Quiz ■ 186
■ Medicare: What Do You Know? ■ 189
■ Do You Know Your Medical Record Rights? ■ 198
■ Do You Know Your Pension Rights? ■ 201
■ Malpractice Suits: Do You Know the Facts from
the Fiction? ■ 208

6 ■ **THE 21 MOST IMPORTANT
HOME MEDICAL TESTS** ■ **213**
■ Body Temperature ■ 215
■ Pulse Measurement and Fitness Testing ■ 216
■ Vision Testing ■ 216
■ Ear Examination ■ 217
■ Self-Exam for Dental Plaque ■ 218
■ Home Blood Pressure Monitoring ■ 218
■ Self-Testing for Lung Function ■ 219
■ Urinalysis ■ 221
■ Self-Testing for Urinary Tract Infections ■ 221
■ Ovulation and Pregnancy Self-Test ■ 222
■ Home Blood Glucose Monitoring ■ 223
■ Home Throat Cultures ■ 223
■ Self-Test for Breath Alcohol ■ 224
■ Home Screening for Bowel Cancer ■ 225
■ Home Test for Pinworms ■ 226
■ Vaginal Self-Exam ■ 226
■ Breast Self-Exam ■ 227
■ Testicular Self-Exam ■ 227

■ Self-Test for Erection Problems ■ 227
■ Sinus Transillumination ■ 228
■ Self-Test for Body Fat Composition ■ 229

BIBLIOGRAPHY ■ **231**

INTRODUCTION

This is a book about you. No, you didn't write it. And it's true, we didn't interview you. But the simple fact is, when you are through using this book, you will probably know more about yourself than you ever did before.

The *People's Medical Society Healthy Body Book* is designed to help you learn more about your health and matters relating to your health. It's a book of questions, questions that will help you determine just what you know—or need to know—about important health issues that confront you daily.

But what good are questions without answers? And that's where you come in. For every question in this book, there is an answer. But not all the answers are found in these pages. Indeed, many of the answers depend on you. What makes you unique is what makes the answers to these questions important.

Nor are all the answers "right" or "wrong." Some of the answers will reveal facts about yourself that you never knew before. Others will help you better understand an issue or subject that has baffled you for years. You might even confirm something you always thought was true, but had no way of verifying.

The *Healthy Body Book* is a book of empowerment. Empowerment is the concept of being able to make decisions on the basis of solid, valid, and relevant information. In health, empowerment is a relatively new concept. Most consumers know little about their medical conditions, the food or medications they may swallow, the training of their practitioners, or even their rights to their own medical record. Most of us have relied on someone else, usually a doctor, to tell us if we are physically fit, are eating the right things, or need to change our life-styles.

What we have done in the *Healthy Body Book* is to create a book of self-tests and quizzes that will empower you with knowledge about yourself and the health-care system. With that knowledge, you will not only become a healthier person, but a smarter consumer of health care.

This book is not designed to replace a physician or other health practitioner. Rather, it is meant to be a guide for your own health and through the health-care system itself. Sadly, many people are using the wrong practitioner for a particular problem simply because they don't know any better. One specific test in this book, "Do You Know What Medical Specialist Does What—and Where," can solve that problem forever.

Many health experts have noted that health is more than not being sick. Being healthy is many things. It is maintaining happiness, reducing stress, being at peace with oneself, and knowing how to find enjoyment out of life. It is having a safe environment, both global and local. It is knowing about your medical care, your doctor, your hospital, and even the home medical tests available to you.

Being healthy and learning about health don't have to be drudgery or a boring task. They don't have to be scary or nerve-racking. Testing yourself about your health and health awareness can be fun and enjoyable. It can also be done in the privacy of your own home—no appointment necessary.

There are two sides to the *Healthy Body Book*. One side is the serious side. Our intention is for you to utilize the tests in these pages to become more enlightened about yourself and health care in general.

The other side is to have fun. And the fun part of this book is taking the fifty-seven different tests wherever and whenever you want to. Take them alone—lock yourself in your attic, where no one will find you, and self-test yourself for hours. Or maybe have a "test-yourself party"—invite some friends over and have them all take the "How to Tell If You're Past Your Prime" test.

You may be wondering where these tests came from. Many have already appeared in magazines or medical publications. They were devised by experts in their fields, and some have been used by practitioners in evaluating their patients.

Other tests were devised specifically for this book. These are the tests dealing with medical rights, practitioners, medical equipment, and insurance. We created them to enlighten and empower you in your quest for maximum health.

Of course, the other question is whether these tests are valid. The answer to that is a resounding yes! We have checked them all. We have verified the answers where factual findings and statements are made. We can assure you that what you read is accurate information at the time of this book's publication.

Finally, why a book like this from the People's Medical Society? As America's largest consumer health advocacy organization, the nonprofit People's Medical Society is dedicated to empowering the medical consumer. Health care in America is the last bastion of nonconsumerism. The idea that consumers can be more involved and active in their own health is our paramount concern. We also believe that you and other medical consumers can understand the factors that make up good health without necessarily having to run to a doctor or hospital for advice. But does that make the People's Medical Society anti-doctor? Of course not! Rather, it makes us pro-consumer. Since its founding in 1983, the People's Medical Society has taken the leadership in helping to bring consumers information they need to be full partners in their health care.

More than 150,000 people have joined the People's Medical Society since its early days. They are the vanguard of a consumer movement committed to improving their health and health-care relationships. They are a "take charge" group of people.

Obviously you, too, are a take-charge type of person or you would not be using this book. We think the *Healthy Body Book* can be an enjoyable way for you to learn more about yourself, your health, and the health-care system. The empowering nature of each test affords you the opportunity to learn at your own speed and in your own way. No lectures, no notes, no bias; the *Healthy Body Book* is your private guide through your world of health.

So this is your book. Have fun using it and learning more about yourself.

≡People's Medical Society®

HEALTHY BODY
▪ B O O K ▪

1. WHO AM I?

W hen we're young, especially in our mid- to late-teen years, we spend a great deal of time trying to find ourselves. We chastise our parents for not understanding us. We search religion and philosophy, trying to find insight into our own character and nature. Sometimes the search for our inner self is successful. And often, just when we find ourselves, we realize that maybe we are not that way anymore. In other words, we realize that we can easily change. It depends on whom and what we encounter.

The five tests that follow are designed to help you get a better understanding of who you are *now*. We think they are a good way to start the book, as they give you a wide range of insight about what makes you who you are.

We start with a test of your overall health. It's called "How to Tell If You're Past Your Prime." We go on to look at what kind of risk taker you are. Then we check your smarts, how loving and understanding you are, and, finally, we show you how to measure the stress in your life.

When you finish these tests, you'll know a lot more about who you are than you did before you began.

HOW TO TELL IF YOU'RE PAST YOUR PRIME: A TEST TO DETERMINE WHETHER YOU'RE OVER THE HILL

Are you reaching your prime? Or have you passed it prematurely? Here is a biological time test designed to help you assess where you really are in your life, physically and mentally.

TEST ONE:
Your Biological Age

You know your chronological age, but what about your biological age? Here's a tailor-made test to tell you.

■ SCORING

1. Start with your present age.
2. Add or subtract the years indicated according to what applies to you.
3. Get a total. Read it and weep—or reform.

Anti-Aging Factors

1. If your blood pressure is 120/80, subtract two years from your age.   −2
2. If your cholesterol is less than 180, subtract one year.   −1
3. If you are in good physical condition, subtract one year.   −1
4. If you have no history of chronic illness, subtract two years.   −2
5. If you have no asthma or respiratory troubles, subtract one year.   −1

6. If your resting pulse rate is less than 60 beats per minute, subtract one year.   −1

7. If you have good vision, subtract one year.   −1

Aging Factors

1. If your blood pressure is over 140/90, add two years to your age.   +2

2. If you are overweight, add three years.   +3

3. If your cholesterol level is greater than 250, add one year.   +1

4. If you smoke more than half a pack a day, add two years.   +2

5. If you have more than two drinks a day, add six months.   +0.5

6. If you have poor post-exercise recovery (it takes a long time for you to regain your stamina), add one year.   +1

7. If you are anemic, add six months.   +0.5

8. If you have poor immunity to infection, add one year.   +1

9. If you suffer from constipation, add one year.   +1

10. If you are chronically fatigued, add one year.   +1

11. If your resting pulse rate is more than 80 beats per minute, add six months.   +0.5

12. If you have a poor short-term memory, add one year.   +1

13. If you have vision problems, add six months.   +0.5

14. If you have sexual difficulties, add six months.   +0.5

TEST TWO:
Your Cardiovascular Age

The health of your heart may best determine how long and how well you'll live, suggest both the International Heart Foundation and the American Heart Association.

■ SCORING

Start this test at zero and check your total against the chart at the end of this test. A high score does not mean you will develop heart disease as you age, but it does mean that there is a potential risk.

Your Age

Getting older increases everyone's chance of suffering heart disease. Anyone older than 55 is likelier to have a heart attack or a stroke than a younger person. There's nothing you can do but consider this factor and count it in.

If you are 56 or older, score one.   1

If you are 55 or younger, score zero.   0

Sex

Men are at a greater risk of cardiovascular complication than women (the occurrence of heart attacks among women is increasing, though).

If you are male, score one.   1

If you are female, score zero.   0

Family History

If you come from a family where there is or has been cardiovascular disease, your chances of being a victim rise—especially if one or more of your close relatives—grandparents, parents, brothers, or sisters—suffered an attack or stroke before 60.

For one or more close blood relatives who have had a heart attack or stroke at or before 60, score twelve.   12

For one or more close blood relatives with a known history of heart disease at or before 60 but no heart attacks or strokes, score ten.   10

For one or more who have had a heart attack or stroke after 60, score six.   6

Otherwise, score zero.   0

Personal History

If you have a history of cardiovascular disease, your chances of more trouble are greater than a nonvictim's.

- If you have had one or more of the following at or before 50—a heart attack, heart or blood vessel surgery, or a stroke—score twenty.   20
- If you have had one or more after 50, score ten.   10
- If you have had none, score zero.   0

Diabetes

Cardiovascular disease runs high among diabetics. If you are a diabetic, check the statement below that applies.

- If you have diabetes before 40 and are now using insulin, score ten.   10
- If you had diabetes at or before 40 and are now using insulin or pills, score five.   5
- If your diabetes is controlled by diet, or your diabetes began after 55, score three.   3
- If you have never had diabetes, score zero.   0

Smoking

- If you smoke two or more packs of cigarettes a day, score ten.   10
- If you smoke between one and two packs a day, or quit smoking less than a year ago, score six.   6
- If you smoke six or more cigars a day or smoke a pipe regularly, score five.   5
- If you smoke less than one pack of cigarettes a day, or quit smoking more than a year ago, score three.   3
- If you smoke less than six cigars a day, or do not inhale a pipe regularly, score three.   3
- If you quit smoking five or more years ago, score one.   1
- If you have never smoked, score zero.   0

Diet

A diet rich in cholesterol and saturated fat gives you a greater risk of heart disease. High cholesterol and triglyceride levels in the blood cause atherosclerotic deposits in the lining of the arteries.

- If you have at least one serving of red meat daily, more than seven eggs a week, and use butter, whole milk, and cheese daily, score eight.   8
- If you eat red meat four to six times a week, eat four to seven eggs a week, use margarine, low-fat dairy products, and some cheese, score four.   4
- If you eat poultry, fish, and a little or no red meat, three or fewer eggs a week, some margarine, and skim-milk products, score zero.   0

Cholesterol

- If your cholesterol level is 276 or higher, score ten.   10
- If it is between 225 and 275, score five.   5
- If it is 224 or below, score zero.   0

High Blood Pressure

When blood pressure goes above normal range and stays there, you have hypertension—meaning your heart must pump harder to get blood through arterial passages. When blood pressure is normal, chances of heart trouble are lower.

- If either number in your blood pressure reading is 160/100 or higher, score ten.   10
- If either number is 140/90 but less than 160/100, score five.   5
- If both numbers are less than 140/90, score zero.   0

Weight

The heavier you are, the more you tip the scales in favor of a heart attack. Is your weight up, down, or on the nose?

Multiply the number of inches you are over 5 feet by five, then add 100 for women and 110 for men. This is your ideal weight in pounds.

If your present weight is more than your ideal weight, subtract your ideal weight from your present weight. This is the amount you are overweight.

- If you are at least 25 pounds overweight, score four.   4
- If you are 10 to 24 pounds overweight, score two.   2
- If you are less than 10 pounds overweight, score zero.   0

Exercise

Physical activity is essential. A lack aggravates heart problems.

- If you engage in any aerobic exercise (brisk walking, jogging, cycling, racquetball, swimming) for more than 15 minutes less than once a week, score four.   4
- If you exercise that hard once or twice a week, score two.   2
- If you engage in that exercise three or more times a week, score zero.   0

Stress

If you are a hurried, harried type who never finds time to enjoy life in the slow lane, you are a more likely candidate for a heart condition.

- If you are frustrated when waiting in line, often in a hurry to complete work or keep appointments, easily angered or irritable, score four.   4
- If you are simply impatient when waiting, occasionally hurried, or are occasionally moody, score two.   2
- If you are relatively comfortable when waiting, seldom rushed, and easygoing, score zero.   0

▪ **SCORING CHART**
HIGH RISK: 40 and above.
MEDIUM RISK: 20–39
LOW RISK: 10 and below.

TEST THREE:

Your Personal Habits, Part I

"You're not getting older, you're getting better," the saying goes. But if you're already pretty good, it can help keep you young. How are your personal habits?

Family

- Do you have open, honest, clear communication? Score one.   1
- Do you have a feeling of self-worth at home? Score one.   1
- Are you flexible about family roles and rules? Score one.   1

Activity

- Do you run, cycle, swim, or walk regularly at least 15 minutes, four times a week? Score three if you do.   3
- If you exercise three times a week, score two.   2
- If you exercise twice a week, score one.   1

Nutrition

- If you eat balanced meals from the four food groups (vegetables, fruits, cereals, and meat or fish), score one.   1
- If you eat breakfast regularly and snack seldom, score one.   1
- If you limit sugar, salt, and junk foods, score one.   1
- If your weight is normal, score one.   1

Toxins

- If you avoid tobacco, marijuana, and needless drugs, and drink less than four cups of coffee or tea a day, score three.   3
- If you're a nonsmoker but drink more than four cups of coffee, score two.   2

Alcohol

- If you take more than two drinks a day, score one.   1
- If you take one or two drinks a day, score two.   2
- If you drink about once a week, score three.   3

Sex, Sleep, and Safety

- If you sleep seven to nine hours a night, score two.   2
- If you are satisfied with your sex life, score two.   2
- If you always wear seat belts in your car, score two.   2

Faith

- If you feel you have a purpose in life, score one.   1
- If you're generally optimistic, score one.   1
- If you can control negative thoughts, score one.   1
- If you're usually relaxed, score three.   3

Intellect

- If you keep reading, learning, and stimulating the mind (nerve cells in the brain that have deteriorated can grow new branches if the mind is stimulated to learn), score one.   1
- If you're always aware of your health and feel responsible for it, score one.   1
- If you can handle anger, guilt, and worry, score one.   1

Career

- If it gives you a sense of direction, score one.   1
- If you find it satisfying, score one.   1
- If you get along well with your boss and coworkers, score one.   1

TEST THREE:

Your Personal Habits, Part II

Add up your score for Part I and multiply by three. Now add or subtract from this score according to your answers to the following questions:

- If all four grandparents lived to age 80, add six.   +6
- If either parent died of a stroke or a heart attack before 50, subtract four.   −4

- If any parent, brother, or sister younger than 50 has (or had) cancer or a heart condition, or has had diabetes since childhood, subtract three.   −3
- If you earn more than $50,000 a year, subtract two.   −2
- If you finished college, add one.   +1
- If you have a graduate or professional degree, add two.   +2
- If you are 65 or older and still working, add three.   +3
- If you work behind a desk, subtract three.   −3
- If your work requires regular, heavy physical labor, add three.   +3
- If you exercise strenuously (tennis, running, swimming, etc.) five times a week for thirty minutes or more, add four; if it's two or three times a week, add two.   +4 or +2
- If you sleep more than ten hours each night, subtract four.   −4
- If you are intense, aggressive, easily angered, subtract three.   −3
- Are you easygoing and relaxed? Add three.   +3
- Are you happy? Add one.   +1
  Unhappy? Subtract three.   −3
- Do you smoke more than two packs a day? Subtract eight.   −8
  One or two? Subtract six.   −6
  One-half to one? Subtract three.   −3
- If you drink the equivalent of a quart of alcohol a day, subtract one.   −1
- Are you overweight by 50 pounds or more? Subtract eight.   −8
  By 30 to 50 pounds? Subtract four.   −4
  By 10 to 30 pounds? Subtract two.   −2
- If you are a woman and see a gynecologist once a year, add two.   +2
- If you are a man older than 40 and have annual checkups, add two.   +2
- If you are between 30 and 40, add two.   +2
- If you are between 50 and 70, add four.   +4
- If you are older than 70, add five.   +5

■ **SCORING**

Tally your final score from Parts I and II of this test to get your life expectancy, according to the chart below.

AVERAGE LIFE EXPECTANCY

SCORE	LIFE EXPECTANCY	
20–29	Male 71.2	Female 77.8
30–39	Male 71.3	Female 77.9
40–49	Male 73.5	Female 78.4
50–59	Male 76.1	Female 79.0
60–69	Male 80.2	Female 83.6
70–79	Male 85.9	Female 87.7
80–90	Male 90.0	Female 91.1

ARE YOU A THRILLAHOLIC?

Take this test and find out . . . .

Fred's money is in savings bonds; Ned's is in penny stocks. Gene goes to the theater on a Friday night; Ed heads for the track. Paul rides a stationary bike for fitness; Chuck races a 500 cc. Honda.

What's going on here?

"Some people simply are born with greater needs for physical excitement and risk than others," stated University of Delaware Professor of psychology Marvin Zuckerman, Ph.D., in *Men's Health*. Thrill seekers may begin to feel downright uncomfortable, Dr. Zuckerman said, if they are forced to put their risk-taking behavior on hold.

Some studies suggest the appetite for excitement may depend on levels of a brain chemical called monoamine oxidase (MAO) inherited at birth. The more MAO we have, the less voltage (i.e., sensory stimulation or risk) it takes to turn us on. Someone like Mario Andretti has very little MAO, the theory goes, while the television character Barney Fife may be drenched in the stuff. The following test should give you an idea of the amount of MAO flowing through you. Simply check the statements that best apply.

1. (a) I would like a job that requires a lot of traveling.
   (b) I would prefer a job in one location.

2. (a) I am invigorated by a brisk, cold day.
   (b) I can't wait to get indoors on a cold day.

3. (a) I get bored seeing the same old faces.
   (b) I like the comfortable familiarity of everyday friends.

4. (a) I would prefer living in an ideal society in which everyone is safe, secure, and happy.
   (b) I would have preferred living in the unsettled days of our history.

5. (a) I sometimes like to do things that are a little frightening.
   (b) A sensible person avoids activities that are dangerous.

6. (a) I would not like to be hypnotized.
   (b) I would like to have the experience of being hypnotized.

7. (a) The most important goal of life is to live it to the fullest and experience as much as possible.
   (b) The most important goal of life is to find peace and happiness.

8. (a) I would like to try parachute jumping.
   (b) I would never want to try jumping out of a plane, with or without a parachute.

9. (a) I enter cold water gradually, giving myself time to get used to the water.
   (b) I like to dive or jump right into the ocean or a cold pool.

10. (a) When I go on vacation, I prefer the comfort of a good room and bed.
    (b) When I go on vacation, I prefer the change of camping out.

11. (a) I prefer people who are emotionally expressive even if they are a bit unstable.
    (b) I prefer people who are emotionally restrained and predictable.

12. (a) A good painting should shock or jolt the senses.
    (b) A good painting should give one a feeling of peace and security.

13. (a) People who ride motorcycles must have some kind of unconscious need to hurt themselves.

   (b) I would like to drive or ride a motorcycle.

■ **SCORING**

Give yourself one point for each of the following statements you checked: 1a, 2a, 3a, 4b, 5a, 6b, 7a, 8a, 9b, 10b, 11a, 12a, 13b. Now tally your score. A high score suggests that you like to live life on the wild side.

0–3: VERY LOW
4–5: LOW
6–9: AVERAGE
10–11: HIGH
12–13: VERY HIGH

Did you score closer to mild than wild?

Don't feel bad. We live in a society that exalts the "courage" it takes to live dangerously, but Dr. Zuckerman says that risks can also be involved in pursuing a career or accepting social and intellectual challenges.

Frank Farley, Ph.D., of the University of Wisconsin, agrees: "Satisfying your curiosity about the world around you, about people and about yourself requires a certain amount of risk."

Some daredevil types, Dr. Zuckerman believes, may be avoiding other "safer" social or intellectual challenges.

So if your idea of a joy ride is shifting positions in your La-Z Boy, relax. You may be a veritable Evel Knievel in your personal or professional life. Thrill seeking also tends to diminish with age, perhaps as we begin to tire of the stuff, so comfort yourself in that.

INTELLIGENCE QUIZ: ARE YOU SMART?

Vanna White has an IQ of 125; Jackie O's is 140. If you're several egg-headed digits behind the stars, not to worry. Only 2 percent of the adult population scores this high; 148 and above is genius category. According to psychologist Howard Gardner of Harvard University's Project Zero, "True intelligence is based on not one but seven categories of smartness."

Edison was a grade-school dropout; Albert Einstein did poorly on standardized tests; Winston Churchill failed English but later went on to win the Nobel Prize for literature.

Conversely, a low IQ score doesn't predict creativity. The two are independent.

The good news is that all of us shine in at least one category, and nobody is a dummy in all seven divisions.

Where does your true intelligence lie? This quiz will tell you where you stand and what to do about it. Read each statement. If it expresses some characteristic of yours and sounds true for the most part, jot down *true*. If it doesn't, mark a *false*. If the statement is sometimes true, sometimes false, leave it blank.

1. I'd rather draw a map than give someone verbal directions.
2. I can play (or used to play) a musical instrument.
3. I can associate music with my moods.
4. I can add or multiply quickly in my head.
5. I like to work with calculators and computers.
6. I pick up new dance steps fast.
7. It's easy for me to say what I think in an argument or debate.
8. I enjoy a good lecture, speech, or sermon.
9. I always know north from south no matter where I am.
10. Life seems empty without music.
11. I always understand the directions that come with new gadgets or appliances.
12. I like to work puzzles and play games.
13. Learning to ride a bike (or skates) was easy.
14. I am irritated when I hear an argument or statement that sounds illogical.
15. My sense of balance and coordination is good.
16. I often see patterns and relationships between numbers faster and easier than others.
17. I enjoy building models (or sculpting).
18. I'm good at finding the fine points of word meanings.

19. I can look at an object one way and see it turned sideways or backward just as easily.
20. I often connect a piece of music with some event in my life.
21. I like to work with numbers and figures.
22. Just looking at shapes of buildings and structures is pleasurable to me.
23. I like to hum, whistle, and sing in the shower or when I'm alone.
24. I'm good at athletics.
25. I'd like to study the structure and logic of languages.
26. I'm usually aware of the expression on my face.
27. I'm sensitive to the expressions on other people's faces.
28. I stay in touch with my moods. I have no trouble identifying them.
29. I am sensitive to the moods of others.
30. I have a good sense of what others think of me.

■ SCORING

If you answered *true* to at least four of the five questions listed in each of the following categories (a) through (e), here's where your abilities lie. Answering *true* to any of the categories (f) through (g) means you have abilities in these areas as well:

   (a) Questions 7, 8, 14, 18, and 25 suggest verbal ability.
   (b) Questions 4, 5, 12, 16, and 21 suggest mathematical ability.
   (c) Questions 2, 3, 10, 20, and 23 suggest musical ability.
   (d) Questions 1, 9, 11, 19, and 22 suggest spatial ability.
   (e) Questions 6, 13, 15, 17, and 24 suggest physical ability.
   (f) Questions 26 and 28 suggest intrapersonal ability (the ability to project yourself, or how you come across to others).
   (g) Questions 27, 29, and 30 suggest interpersonal ability (sensitivity to others).

THE LOVE AND UNDERSTANDING QUIZ

Love means never having to tell a lie. Or does it? Should you always be totally honest with your husband or wife? Or are some things better left unsaid? Test your intimacy skills: Here are ten dilemmas that might confront you someday. What's the most loving and understanding thing to do? Compare your responses to the advice of top marriage counselors and psychologists. (The following quiz by Morton Hunt is reprinted from *Redbook*.)

Do you always tell your husband or wife the truth, the whole truth, and nothing but the truth? Are you totally honest and self-revealing about your feelings, thoughts, and experiences? Should you be?

Many young couples believe—and some marriage counselors would agree with them—that the secret to a good marriage is good communication, by which they mean telling each other absolutely everything. These couples feel that to withhold information is to create a barrier to intimacy, which is the key to marital success.

Other couples, however—and other marriage counselors—believe that we owe it to the person we love to conceal or even lie about some of the things we feel and think—or have done. These people would argue that telling a lie is sometimes more loving and understanding than telling the truth. Says Karl E. Scheibe, Ph.D., professor of psychology at Wesleyan University in Middletown, Connecticut, who has done research on lying and truth telling, "Love is not built on lies, but it does include tact, kindness, and protection of the other—and this sometimes precludes telling the truth. Some lies embody a larger truth—the truth of caring."

Which side is right? And how is a husband or wife to decide what to reveal and what to conceal? Seeking clarifying principles, author Morton Hunt presented ten hypothetical situations to a panel of eight marriage counselors, psychiatrists, and psychologists, and asked their opinions on how each situation would best be handled. Although the panel members were not always unanimous in their responses, in most cases the majority of them did answer similarly—and for similar reasons. Here are the ten situations and the panel's enlightening, and often surprising, comments.

1. Artie, boyish and exuberant, tends to drink too much around
   others and then becomes somewhat loud and behaves a little
   foolishly. This embarrasses his wife, Bobbie, who also fears that
   her husband's behavior will have a negative effect on their friendships. She should
   (a) Talk to her husband about her feelings.
   (b) Keep quiet and let him enjoy himself.

In one way or another, all of our panelists say that, when considering whether or not to tell a truth that will hurt someone, the first
question to ask is whether telling can benefit the person who will be
hurt. Says family sociologist and marriage and family therapist
Graham B. Spanier, Ph.D., "Communication is appropriate when
change is possible or when the problem can be solved; it is not
appropriate when change is not possible or no solution to the problem is likely."

Presuming, then, that Artie is not an alcoholic and can control his
party behavior, Bobbie should tell him that he is behaving in a way
that she finds embarrassing. But how and when she tells him is
crucial. Laura J. Singer, Ed.D., a marital therapist, advises, "She
should mention her concerns delicately and see how he reacts. He
may not be aware of the way he is being viewed by others, and
changing his behavior may not be a big deal to him."

Bernice Hunt, M.S., a certified clinical mental health counselor
and marital therapist in Millwood and East Hampton, New York,
and wife of author Hunt, suggests that Bobbie start her conversation with a positive statement such as, "I love you and enjoy your
boyish exuberance, but . . ." Then she can specify how she'd like
Artie to act. "Instead of attacking his current behavior," says Hunt,
"Bobbie could say something like, 'I have much more fun with you
at parties when you limit your drinking so that you remain the
Artie I know and love.' " Hunt feels that telling Artie about his
behavior will not only benefit him, but will prevent possible future
damage to the marriage: "If Bobbie fails to tell him, her resentment
will build up, and this is bound to erode their relationship."

Several other panelists add that Bobbie should tell Artie only when he's in a good mood and is able to handle criticism. "Bobbie should choose the best time and place to bring up the subject," says Ellen Berman, M.D., marital therapist and associate professor of psychiatry at the University of Pennsylvania, and senior consultant to the Marriage Council of Philadelphia. "Right before going to a party, for example, is not the time to begin such a discussion."

2. Charles is short and, though only 32, balding and roly-poly. At the beach, he notices that his wife, Doris, keeps looking at a tall, slim young man with a thick head of hair. Trying to sound light-hearted, Charles says to her, "Turns you on, doesn't he? Bet you wish I looked like that." He's right, she does. What should she do?
   (a) Admit it.
   (b) Deny it.

This situation seems trivial, but may not be. Charles may be expressing his insecurity and low self-esteem, and the truth is just what he doesn't need to hear. But even if he's quite inwardly se- cure, Doris probably shouldn't tell the whole truth. Clifford Sager, M.D., director of family psychiatry at the Jewish Board of Family and Children's Services, and clinical professor of psychiatry at the New York Hospital-Cornell Medical Center, both in New York City, says, "Every person is entitled to have private thoughts, especially if these thoughts are critical of something his or her spouse can't do anything about."

Moreover, Doris may not only be admiring the young man's looks but also momentarily imagining herself making love with him. If so, she definitely should keep quiet. Says Frederick G. Humphrey, Ed.D., past president of the American Association for Marriage and Family Therapy, "Doris has a right to enjoy her fantasies—but privately. Revealing one's sexual fantasies about other people can be overwhelming to one's partner." And it's selfish—it gratifies the teller of the fantasy but ignores the partner's need to believe that he or she is still desired exclusively.

Most of our experts point out, however, that since Charles *could* do something about his weight, it would be legitimate for Doris to admit the part of her thoughts that touches upon her husband's weight. "The important question in such situations isn't simply whether to tell the truth or not, but what *part* to tell," says Diane Sollee, M.S.W., a marital and family therapist in Washington, D.C., and director of communications for the American Association for Marriage and Family Therapy. "Doris could, and probably should, say something about Charles's weight—something loving, like 'I'd like it if you were slim, too, because I want to have you around for a long while.' "

Whether to reveal even this much of what she is thinking depends on the quality of Charles and Doris's relationship, says Dr. Berman. "If Charles and Doris have a great relationship and enjoy good sex, she might not admit the whole truth but could tell him a reassuring version of it in the form of a joke such as, 'I like to window-shop, but I only buy the best—and that's you.' But if Charles is indirectly saying that the marriage hasn't been going well and that he's feeling bad about more than his looks, Doris has to decide if this is the time to talk about her dissatisfactions. If he needs reassurance, she should kiss him and change the subject."

Several of our experts offered one final word of caution: Doris should not tell Charles the truth if she's currently feeling angry at him. Telling a spouse a painful truth in anger might be a way to hurt him and get even, but it will do nothing to resolve the source of that anger.

3. Edith and Frank have been married for five years. As time has passed, she has had to admit to herself that Frank isn't as intelligent as she thought, and that he's definitely less intelligent than she. In their arguments about politics, how best to invest their savings, and many other matters, he often angrily says, "You obviously think I'm not very bright—not half as bright as you." She should
   (a) Admit it.
   (b) Deny it.

Our panel is virtually unanimous: Edith should deny it; to admit her thoughts would humiliate Frank and damage his pride to no good end, since he can't do anything to increase his intelligence.

But denying what she feels won't make the problem go away. "Edith may need to learn how to balance Frank's redeeming qualities and special talents against his intellectual shortcomings," says Hunt. "If she can't do that, we may have to examine, with the help of a therapist, whether she made a mistake and ought to end the marriage."

Dr. Singer adds that Edith should look at how she is contributing to Frank's feelings of inferiority. "Edith may be saying certain things that call attention to those aspects of his intellect that are less developed. She may be ignoring areas in which he is more competent than she."

Dr. Berman feels that Edith should also change some of her own old-fashioned preconceptions. "Edith should ask herself why it bothers her that she's smarter than her husband in certain areas," says Dr. Berman. "There's no rule that a man has to be intellectually superior to a woman in everything."

4. The day before her 34th birthday, Grace studies herself in the mirror—the fine lines around her eyes and the slight sag of her breasts fill her with despair. Her husband, Howard, walks into the bedroom and sees the look on her face. "What's wrong?" he asks. "What's troubling you?" She should
   (a) Tell him the truth.
   (b) Tell him some innocuous lie.

Our panelists all agree that Grace should tell Howard the truth, provided he isn't currently under some severe pressure that might make him unable to respond to her with sensitivity and compassion—and provided, too, that Grace knows him to be generally caring and kind. If Howard is the kind of man who habitually makes fun of other people's frailties, Grace should *not* tell him the truth, for in doing so she might only be opening herself up to needless hurt. If that's the kind of man he is, and he can't be changed—and she is nonetheless committed to the marriage—lying will not only protect her feelings but also protect their relationship.

If, on the other hand, Howard is the kind of man who will respond to Grace's insecurities with compassion and reassurance, telling the truth will benefit both of them. "Howard needs to know that Grace needs some special recognition as she begins to struggle with the normal aging process," says Dr. Humphrey. If she does not tell him how she feels, she shuts him out at a time when she needs him; telling him draws them closer.

"Concealing a fear about one's self interferes with intimacy," says Dr. Sager. "But if Grace can tell Howard her fears, she'll establish an additional bond between them. They will then become collaborators in dealing with the problem. For example, he may say, 'Are you asking me about plastic surgery?' and help her make a decision for or against it. Or he may reassure her by saying, 'Come off it! I love you! And I'm balder than I used to be, and you love me. We're going to keep getting older—and loving each other.' "

5. Irv was not terribly sexual even when he and Janice were newlyweds. Now, seven years later, though they're only in their mid-thirties, he's rarely interested in sex. When she approaches him, he's usually either not in the mood or unable to perform. Apologetically, he blames his lack of interest on career worries and too much work, then adds, "I'll bet you wish you had married somebody sexier." He's right; she often wonders what sex would be like with another man. She should
   (a) Admit it.
   (b) Deny it.

All of our panelists agree that because Irv and Janice are still young, Irv's low sex drive may very well stem from some correctable physical or emotional problem—perhaps a problem existing in the marriage itself. And because his low sex drive troubles both spouses in different ways, the problem, if ignored, could drive them apart and make them both vulnerable to outside temptation.

For this reason, Dr. Scheibe would urge the couple to begin talking alone together about the problem; talking may be enough in itself to solve the difficulties. For example, Janice could reply to Irv's comment by saying, "Yes, sometimes I'd like to have sex more often than we do now. I'd like it if you were more aggressive. But sex is not the only thing in life, and it's certainly not why we got married. It is a problem, but one we can live with—and live with better if we are honest with each other about our feelings." This might enable them to start working toward a compromise: perhaps a bit more sexual responsiveness on Irv's part and a bit less sexual pressure from Janice—if, indeed, she *is* pressuring Irv. The result could be less stress for both of them.

Dr. Spanier emphasizes, however, that Janice should not merely vent her grievance. "Telling the truth just to get something off your chest is rarely productive," he says, "unless it leads to a calm, intelligent, mutually supportive discussion of the issues. Without such a discussion, Irv and Janice will find their relationship growing worse. A therapist may be able to help them resolve their problem in a constructive way, but the essential first step is for Janice to speak up."

Several panelists also suggested that perhaps Irv needs to be encouraged to examine his priorities. If his lack of sex drive is in fact due to overwork and fatigue, and not caused by some physical problem, he may be putting too high a value on professional success and too low a value on the joys of marital satisfaction.

6. When they're with other people, Ken brags incessantly about himself and his accomplishments. His wife, Louise, feels ashamed of him when he behaves this way; she fears it will make them unpopular. She should
   (a) Tell him.
   (b) Keep it to herself.

Most of our panelists feel that, because Ken might be able to control his boastfulness if he were made aware of it, Louise ought to tell him gently how she feels. Says Dr. Scheibe, "One of the things a spouse is for is to tell you when you've got spinach caught in your teeth." Louise also needs to talk to Ken to prevent the erosion of her own feelings toward him. "If she wants to stay happily married to him, she'll have to bite the bullet and confront him—lovingly but firmly," says Dr. Humphrey.

But several of these experts also warn that telling Ken the truth may not help him. It's possible that his bragging actually masks deep-seated insecurities, and this may make it impossible for him to hear and accept Louise's criticism. Indeed, his problem may be one that can only be helped through therapy—in which case Louise may have to keep quiet and try to accept her husband as he is unless he decides to seek help. "A wife can't play therapist for her husband," says Dr. Sager, "and she shouldn't attempt to explore his insecurities. That's a job for someone outside the relationship."

Dr. Singer agrees. In her opinion, if a problem is "interactive"—meaning that it is a problem between the two spouses—a husband or wife should speak out. But if, as in this case, the problem is "intrapsychic"—meaning that the problem exists within one spouse and has nothing to do with that spouse's partner—then it is usually better for the partner to say nothing. "Ken needs to develop a stronger sense of self and become less dependent on the rewards of narcissistic behavior," says Dr. Singer. "Since Louise can't help him do that, she should keep quiet."

Essentially then, our panelists agree that, in this case, Louise's decision to tell or not to tell should depend on how superficial or deep-seated she feels Ken's problem is. If she feels it's only a matter of easily correctable style, she should tell him—for his good as well as hers. If she feels, however, that his bragging is a symptom of a deeper, more basic personality problem, she should keep quiet. If Louise does decide that Ken's problem runs deeper, she may also begin to question whether she wants to remain married to him. To counterbalance those doubts, our experts recommend that she ask herself what attracted her to him initially and which of his qualities outweigh his insecurity. Those qualities are still there.

7. Michael is a gentle, rather timid man. His meekness, when sales-
   people and repairmen fail to provide adequate service, or when
   his boss mistreats him, drives his wife, Nancy, wild. She's sad-
   dened for his sake and humiliated for her own. What should she
   do?
   (a) Tell him how she feels.
   (b) Keep her feelings to herself.

Half of our panelists agree that, because Michael may be able to
change, Nancy could tell him, gently and supportively, how she
feels. Scorn or criticism, however, would be hurtful not only to him,
but to their relationship as well. And if she tries to tell him how he
should act—"Why don't you fight back when that happens? What
are you afraid of?"—she will only make things worse. If Nancy
can't accept Michael as he is, she has to open a discussion of his
behavior tactfully and kindly—perhaps by suggesting that they go
into assertiveness training together.

Dr. Berman points out, however, that Michael may refuse to see
his behavior as a problem. "If so, Nancy will have to learn to live
with it." Michael may be right: Nancy may be a traditional woman
who expects her man to be aggressive, while Michael simply may
not be cut from the traditional cloth. If this is the case, Nancy will
have to work on changing herself rather than on changing him.
"Nancy may need to reexamine her own feelings about stereotypi-
cal gender behavior," says Dr. Sager. "She may never have looked
closely at her own expectation that a man should be tough. The
problem may simply be hers, not Michael's."

Several of our experts add that, even if Michael is overly timid,
the timidity is his problem—an "intrapsychic" problem—*not* a problem between *them* and that, therefore, Nancy should keep quiet.

8. Olivia's fiancé, whom she adored, died in a car accident, and it
   has taken her four years to get over his death. Now Olivia is
   involved with a divorced man named Paul, and she is thinking of
   marrying him. Because his first marriage failed, Paul is feeling
   rather insecure. One night, after making love, he asks Olivia,

"Do you love me as much as you loved him?" The truth, alas, is no. Olivia's love for Paul is calmer and more sedate. She should
(a) Tell him and explain.
(b) Lie.

Our panelists all agree that Olivia should tell the truth and explain. None of them are advising, however, that Olivia admit she loved her fiancé more. Instead, they recommend that she say something about how the two loves are different and can't be compared. Such an answer is, in effect, an evasion, but in this case evasion or deception is the kind and protective choice. It strengthens Paul's shaky self-confidence and gives their love a chance to grow.

Says Dr. Scheibe, "Olivia doesn't have to accept the premise of Paul's question—that one love can be compared to another. Instead, she might say something like 'Time passes, circumstances are different.' " Dr. Singer agrees. "The only way to help him and the relationship is to say, 'I love you differently. I'm four years older, and I have been through a terrible trauma. I'm a different person than I was four years ago.' " Dr. Sager feels that Paul's question is truly irrelevant. "But Olivia should reassure him by stressing that this is *another* love, and by talking openly about her previous relationship without making any comparisons between the two."

Says Bernice Hunt, "To help Paul—and to help their relationship—Olivia should reply that no two loves are alike, that each has its special aspects and rewards, and that a new love is *different* from, not more or less than, an earlier one. Olivia should also be aware that no one can predict how a relationship will develop over time—this one could eventually become far more dear to her than her last love was." Hunt's comments have special significance to me: We married after her beloved husband—who was a friend of mine—died of leukemia. We've been happily married for sixteen years.

9. After nine years, Regina feels that her marriage to Sam has grown unaccountably dull. She can't put her finger on any particular problem, and she doesn't think Sam is at fault in any way, but she's depressed that their married life has become so joyless

for no reason. Sam senses her mood and asks her what's wrong.
She should
(a) Tell him how she feels.
(b) Tell him a white lie.

All of the panelists say that it is essential for Regina to tell Sam
how she feels, because, even though she can't pinpoint the problem,
a problem obviously *does* exist. Only by talking honestly together
can they hope to find it.

Once identified, the problem may prove to be not all that serious
or hard to deal with. Says Dr. Sager, "It might be that their early
passion has merely given way to the quieter bonding of a long-term
relationship, and that Regina hasn't come to terms with this. Or it
may be that they have drifted into deadening routines and are
forgetting to show each other affection and do interesting things
together. In either case, talking about Regina's dissatisfaction may
lead to useful action."

Dr. Singer recommends that Regina gently tell Sam how she
feels. Then, together, they can try to identify the problem and come
up with a solution. "Regina might suggest, for example, that they
go away together for a few days of pure fun and relaxation. Then,
when they return, they can try to keep some of that spirit of fun
alive in their daily lives. Regina should also ask herself what she
may need to change about herself in order to make the marriage
more stimulating and enjoyable."

Some of our panelists warn, however, that grave difficulties may
be lurking below the surface dullness of this couple's marriage. "It's
absolutely critical that Regina say something to Sam because her
depression and appraisal of the marriage as 'joyless' suggest that
something is seriously wrong," says Dr. Berman. Her only hope for
motivating her husband to join her in searching out and working on
the problem is to tell him how she feels. Keeping her dissatisfaction
to herself may doom the marriage.

10. While her husband, Ted, is away on a month-long business trip
    in Europe, a man Ursula had a wild affair with in her college

days comes to town and calls her—for old time's sake. They meet and, to Ursula's astonishment, end up in bed. Afterward, she tells herself that the tryst was a stupid, impulsive thing to do and that it won't affect her marriage. But she cannot rid herself of a nagging sense of guilt. When Ted comes home, she finds herself yearning to tell him about the episode and beg his forgiveness. She should

(a) Tell him.

(b) Keep quiet.

The panelists are in almost unanimous agreement: Ursula should say nothing. "Telling Ted could be devastating to him," says Dr. Spanier. "Assuming this was an episodic affair with no promise of continuing commitment and no potential aftershocks that could complicate the marriage, Ursula should keep it to herself."

Ursula may find it extremely painful to remain silent, but our panelists say that this is her problem—unloading the secret to relieve herself of guilt would only hurt Ted and their relationship. Says Dr. Singer, "What could she possibly gain by confessing the affair? She would simply make Ted suffer while assuaging her guilt. It would be different if the affair were a threat to the marriage, but it's not. So no good will come from unloading her baggage on his back."

Diane Sollee points out that keeping a hurtful truth to one's self is often the *mature* way to act. "If you have to confess everything to your partner, you're being totally dependent," she says. "You're saying that you feel safe only when your partner knows everything about you and takes responsibility for deciding how to handle any problems. But if you are your own person, you take responsibility for deciding either to tell or to withhold a piece of information."

A number of panelists add that if Ursula cannot endure the guilt, she should unburden herself to a trustworthy third party—such as a dear friend, a minister, or a therapist—who will not be damaged by her confession and who can help her sort through her feelings. Says Dr. Humphrey, "Only after more exploration can Ursula figure out what would be best for *her* and for *them*."

Sollee adds, however, that, in this era of AIDS and other sexually transmitted diseases, there may indeed be an overriding reason for Ursula to tell Ted about the affair. "Unless she and her sex partner practiced safe sex," says Sollee, "by *not* telling, she may be endangering her husband's life."

Ursula could, of course, be tested for the AIDS virus before deciding whether to confess. Unfortunately, it can take up to six months, or longer, for the antibodies that indicate exposure to the disease to show up in the blood. If Ursula and Ted have any kind of regular sex life, it would be difficult for her to avoid sex with Ted for that long without doing as much damage to their relationship as she risks doing by telling him the truth.

The break with traditional sex roles that took place in the 1960s and 1970s led many couples to believe that it is necessary for them to be totally honest with each other. Marriage is now supposed to be a partnership between equals, and real intimacy between equals can only be achieved, they reason, when both partners open their hearts to each other, holding nothing back.

At first, many therapists and marriage counselors supported the idea. But their experience working with couples has caused many experts to change their minds. These specialists now believe—as do our panelists—that concealing or lying about certain thoughts, feelings, and facts can sometimes be the wiser, more loving, more understanding, and more marriage-sustaining course of action. Intimacy, we now know, means confiding and sharing—but not totally. Out of love for our partner, and to preserve our marital relationship, we should keep some things to ourselves.

STRESS RATING SCALE

Researchers at the University of Washington School of Medicine developed this scale for ranking stressful events in a person's life.

The higher the total score accumulated in the preceding year, the more likely there will be a serious illness in the immediate future.

EVENT	VALUE
Death of spouse	100
Divorce	73
Marital separation	65
Jail term	63
Death of close family member	63
Personal injury or illness	53
Marriage	50
Fired from work	47
Marital reconciliation	45
Retirement	45
Change in family member's health	44
Pregnancy	40
Sex difficulties	39
Addition to family	39
Business readjustment	39
Change in financial status	38
Death of close friend	37
Change to different line of work	36
Change in number of marital arguments	36
Mortgage or loan over $10,000	31
Foreclosure of mortgage or loan	30
Change in work responsibilities	29
Son or daughter leaving home	29
Trouble with in-laws	29
Outstanding personal achievement	28
Spouse begins or stops work	26
Starting or finishing school	26
Change in living conditions	25
Revision of personal habits	24
Trouble with boss	23
Change in work hours, conditions	20
Change in residence	20
Change in schools	20
Change in recreational habits	19
Change in church activities	19
Change in social activities	18
Mortgage or loan under $10,000	17

EVENT	VALUE
Change in sleeping habits	16
Change in number of family gatherings	15
Change in eating habits	15
Vacation	13
Christmas season	12
Minor violation of the law	11

2. YOU ARE WHAT YOU EAT!

As science learns more about nutrition and its impact on health, the almost whimsical line "You are what you eat!" takes on more seriousness.

Over the last few decades, we have gained a far greater understanding of the effects certain types of foods have on our well-being. We know that too much fat in the diet is related to elevated risks of heart disease. We know that certain vitamins are necessary at certain levels to help our bodies function in certain ways.

With all the knowledge we have gained about diet and nutrition, along with the speed at which it is being passed along to us, it is no wonder many people are confused. What can I eat today? What was wrong with what I had yesterday? Am I too fat? Is my sodium intake too high or too low?

The nine tests that follow are designed to help you cut through the confusion. Not only do they reveal your knowledge of diet and nutritional matters, but they also help teach you important facts about the foods you eat.

By the time you have finished this chapter, you will know more about your own nutrition than you ever did before. But more importantly, you are going to find out ways you can improve yourself through the foods you eat.

HOW'S YOUR DIET?*

The forty-two questions below will help you focus on the key features of your diet. The (+) or (−) numbers under/next to each set of answers instantly pat you on the back for good habits or alert you to problems you may not even realize you have. (Sorry.)

The Grand Total rates your overall diet, on a scale from "Super" to "Arghh!"

The quiz focuses on fat, sodium, sugar, fiber, and vitamins A and C. It doesn't attempt to cover everything in your diet. Also, it doesn't attempt to measure precisely how much of these key nutrients you eat.

What the quiz *will do* is give you a rough sketch of your current eating habits and imply what you can do to improve them.

Finally, please don't despair over a less-than-perfect score. A healthy diet isn't built overnight.

■ INSTRUCTIONS

- Under each answer is a number with a + or − sign in front of it. Circle the number that is directly beneath the answer you choose. That's your score for the question.
- Circle only one number for each question, unless the instructions tell you to "average two or more scores if necessary."

* Pages 32–49 are Copyright 1989, Center for Science in the Public Interest. Reprinted from *Nutrition Action Healthletter* (1501 Sixteenth Street, N.W., Washington, DC 20036-1499. $19.95 for 10 issues).

- How to average. In answering question 19, for example, if you drink fruit juice (+1) and coffee (−1) on a typical day, add the two scores (which gives you 0) and then divide by 2. That gives you a score of 0 for that question. If averaging gives you a fraction, round it off to the nearest whole number.
- Make sure you pay attention to serving sizes. For example, a serving of vegetables is 1/2 cup. If you usually eat one cup of vegetables at a time, count it as two servings.
- Add up all your + scores, and write the resulting figure in the Total (+) column at the end of the quiz.
- Add up all your − scores, and write the resulting figure in the Total (−) column at the end of the quiz.
- Subtract the Total (−) column from the Total (+) column. That will give you your Grand Total.

QUIZ

1. How many times per week do you eat unprocessed red meat (steak, roast beef, lamb or pork chops, burgers, etc.)?
   (a) 1 or less   +3
   (b) 2–3   +2
   (c) 4–5   −1
   (d) 6 or more   −3
2. After cooking, how large is the serving of red meat you usually eat? (To convert from raw to cooked, reduce by 25 percent. For example, 4 ounces of raw meat shrinks to 3 ounces after cooking. There are 16 ounces in a pound.)
   (a) 8 ounces or more   −3
   (b) 6–7 ounces   −1
   (c) 4–5 ounces   +1
   (d) 3 ounces or less   +3
   (e) don't eat red meat   +3
3. Do you trim the visible fat when you cook or eat red meat?
   (a) yes   +3
   (b) no   −3
   (c) don't eat red meat   +3

4. How many times per week do you eat processed meats (hot dogs, bacon, sausage, bologna, luncheon meats, etc.)?
(a) none   +3
(b) less than 1   +2
(c) 1–2   0
(d) 3–4   −1
(e) 5 or more   −3

5. What kind of ground meat or poultry do you usually eat?
(a) regular ground beef   −3
(b) lean ground beef   −2
(c) extra-lean ground beef   −1
(d) ground round   0
(e) ground turkey   +1
(f) don't eat   +3

6. What type of bread do you usually eat?
(a) whole wheat or other whole grain   +3
(b) rye   +2
(c) pumpernickel   +2
(d) white, "wheat," French, or Italian   −2

7. How many times per week do you eat deep-fried foods (fish, chicken, vegetables, potatoes, etc.)?
(a) none   +3
(b) 1–2   0
(c) 3–4   −1
(d) 5 or more   −3

8. How many servings of vegetables do you eat per day? (One serving = 1/2 cup. Include nonfried potatoes.)
(a) none   −3
(b) 1   0
(c) 2   +1
(d) 3   +2
(e) 4 or more   +3

9. How many servings of cruciferous vegetables do you usually eat per week? (Count *only* kale, broccoli, cauliflower, cabbage,

Brussels sprouts, greens, bok choy, kohlrabi, turnip, and ruta-
baga. One serving = 1/2 cup.)
(a) none   −3
(b) 1–3   +1
(c) 4–6   +2
(d) 7 or more   +3

10. How many servings of vitamin-A-rich fruits or vegetables do
you usually eat per week? (Count *only* carrots, pumpkin, sweet
potatoes, cantaloupe, spinach, winter squash, greens, apricots,
and broccoli. One serving = 1/2 cup.)
(a) none   −3
(b) 1–3   +1
(c) 4–6   +2
(d) 7 or more   +3

11. How many times per week do you eat at a fast-food restaurant?
(Include burgers, fried fish or chicken, croissant or biscuit sandwiches, topped potatoes, and other main dishes. Omit meals of
just plain baked potato, broiled chicken, or salad.)
(a) none   +3
(b) less than 1   +1
(c) 1   0
(d) 2   −1
(e) 3   −2
(f) 4 or more   −3

12. How many servings of grains rich in complex carbohydrates do
you eat per day? (One serving = 1 slice of bread, 1 large pancake,
or 1/2 cup cooked cereal, rice, pasta, bulgur, wheat berries,
kasha, or millet. Omit heavily sweetened cold cereals.)
(a) none   −3
(b) 1–2   0
(c) 3–4   +1
(d) 5–6   +2
(e) 7 or more   +3

13. How many servings of beer, wine, or liquor do you drink?

(Count as one serving: 12 ounces regular or light beer, 4 ounces wine, or 1 ounce liquor.)

(a) 1 or less a week   +3

(b) 2–3 a week   +1

(c) 4–7 a week   0

(d) 2 a day   −2

(e) more than 2 a day   −3

14. How many times per week do you eat fish or shellfish? (Omit deep-fried items, tuna packed in oil, shrimp, squid, and mayonnaise-laden tuna salad—a little mayo is okay.)

(a) none   −2

(b) 1–2   +1

(c) 3–4   +2

(d) 5 or more   +3

15. How many times per week do you eat cheese? (Include pizza, cheeseburgers, veal or eggplant parmigiana, cream cheese, etc. Omit low-fat or "lite" cheeses.)

(a) 1 or less   +3

(b) 2–3   +2

(c) 4–5   −1

(d) 6 or more   −3

16. How many servings of fresh fruit do you consume per day?

(a) none   −3

(b) 1   0

(c) 2   +1

(d) 3   +2

(e) 4 or more   +3

17. Do you remove the skin before eating poultry?

(a) yes   +3

(b) no   −3

(c) don't eat poultry   +3

18. What do you usually put on your bread or toast? (Average two or more scores if necessary.)

(a) butter   −3

(b) cream cheese   −3

(c) margarine   −2

(d) diet margarine   −1

(e) jam   0

(f) fruit butter   +3

(g) nothing   +3

19. Which of these beverages do you drink on a typical day? (Average two or more scores if necessary.)

(a) fruit juice   +1

(b) water or club soda   +3

(c) diet soda   −1

(d) coffee or tea   −1

(e) soda or fruit drink or ade   −3

20. How many servings of caffeine-containing beverages do you drink per day? (One serving = 1 cup of coffee or tea, or 12 ounces of cola.)

(a) none   +3

(b) 1   +1

(c) 2   −1

(d) 3   −2

(e) 4 or more   −3

21. Which flavorings do you most frequently add to your foods? (Average two or more scores if necessary.)

(a) garlic or lemon juice   +3

(b) herbs or spices   +3

(c) soy sauce   −2

(d) margarine   −2

(e) salt   −3

(f) butter   −3

(g) nothing   +3

22. What do you eat most frequently as a snack? (Average two or more scores if necessary.)

(a) fruits or vegetables   +3

(b) sweetened yogurt   +2

(c) nuts   −1

(d) chips   −2

(e) cookies   −2

(f) granola bar   −2

(g) candy bar   −3

(h) pastry   −3

(i) nothing   0

23. What is your most typical breakfast? (Subtract an extra 3 points if you also eat bacon or sausage.)

(a) croissant, Danish, or doughnut   −3

(b) eggs   −3

(c) pancakes or waffles   −2

(d) nothing   0

(e) cereal or bread   +3

(f) yogurt or cottage cheese   +3

24. What do you usually eat for dessert?

(a) pie, pastry, or cake   −3

(b) ice cream   −3

(c) yogurt, ice milk, or sorbet   +1

(d) fruit   +3

(e) nothing   +3

25. How many times per week do you eat beans, split peas, or lentils?

(a) none   −2

(b) 1   +1

(c) 2   +2

(d) 3 or more   +3

26. What kind of milk do you drink?

(a) whole   −3

(b) 2% low-fat   −1

(c) 1% low-fat   +2

(d) ½ % or skim   +3

(e) none   0

27. What dressings or toppings do you usually add to your salads? (*Add* two or more scores if necessary.)

(a) nothing, lemon, or vinegar   +3

(b) reduced-calorie dressing   +1

(c) regular dressing   −1

(d) croutons or bacon bits   −1

(e) cole slaw, pasta salad, or potato salad   −1

28. What sandwich fillings do you eat most frequently? (Average two or more scores if necessary.)
    (a) luncheon meat   −3
    (b) cheese or roast beef   −1
    (c) peanut butter   0
    (d) tuna, salmon, chicken, or turkey   +3
29. What do you usually spread on your sandwiches? (Average two or more scores if necessary.)
    (a) mayonnaise   −2
    (b) light mayonnaise   −1
    (c) mustard   0
    (d) catsup   0
    (e) nothing   +3
30. How many egg yolks do you eat per week? (Add 1 yolk for every slice of quiche you eat.)
    (a) 2 or less   +3
    (b) 3–4   +2
    (c) 5–6   +1
    (d) 7 or more   −3
31. How many times per week do you eat canned or dried soups? (Omit low-sodium, low-fat soups.)
    (a) none   +3
    (b) 1–2   0
    (c) 3–4   −2
    (d) 5 or more   −3
32. How many servings of a rich source of calcium do you eat per day? (One serving = 2/3 cup milk or yogurt, 1 ounce cheese, 1 1/2 ounces sardines, 3 1/2 ounces salmon, 5 ounces tofu, 1 cup greens or broccoli, or 200 mg of a calcium supplement.)
    (a) none   −3
    (b) 1   +1
    (c) 2   +2
    (d) 3 or more   +3
33. What do you usually order on your pizza? (Nonmeat toppings include green pepper, mushrooms, onions, and other vegetables. Subtract 1 extra point if you order extra cheese.)

(a) no cheese w/nonmeat toppings   +3

(b) cheese w/nonmeat toppings   +1

(c) cheese   0

(d) cheese w/meat toppings   −3

(e) don't eat pizza   +2

34. What kind of cookies do you usually eat?

(a) graham crackers   +1

(b) ginger snaps   +1

(c) oatmeal   −1

(d) chocolate coated, chocolate chip, or peanut butter   −3

(e) sandwich cookies (like Oreos)   −3

(f) don't eat cookies   +3

35. What kind of frozen dessert do you usually eat? (Subtract 1 extra point for each topping—whipped cream, hot fudge, nuts, etc.)

(a) gourmet ice cream   −3

(b) regular ice cream   −1

(c) sorbet, sherbet, or ices   +1

(d) frozen yogurt or ice milk   +1

(e) don't eat frozen desserts   +3

36. What kind of cake or pastry do you usually eat?

(a) cheesecake, pie, or any microwave cake   −3

(b) cake with frosting or filling   −2

(c) cake without frosting   −1

(d) angel food cake   +1

(e) unfrosted muffin, banana bread, or carrot cake   0

(f) don't eat cakes or pastries   +3

37. How many times per week does your dinner contain grains, vegetables, or beans, but little or no animal protein (meat, poultry, fish, eggs, milk, or cheese)?

(a) none   −1

(b) 1   +1

(c) 2   +2

(d) 3   +3

38. Which of the following salty snacks do you typically eat?

(a) potato chips or packaged popcorn   −3

(b) tortilla chips   −1

(c) light potato chips   −2

(d) salted pretzels   −1

(e) unsalted pretzels   +1

(f) homemade air-popped popcorn   +3

(g) don't eat   +3

39. What do you usually use to sauté vegetables or other foods? (Vegetable oil includes safflower, corn, canola, olive, sunflower, and soybean.)

(a) butter or lard   −3

(b) more than 1 tablespoon of margarine or vegetable oil   −1

(c) no more than 1 tablespoon of margarine or vegetable oil   +1

(d) water or broth   +3

40. What kind of cereal do you usually eat?

(a) hot whole-grain (like oatmeal or Wheatena)   +3

(b) cold whole-grain (like Shredded Wheat)   +3

(c) cold low-fiber (like corn flakes)   0

(d) sugary cold low-fiber (like Frosted Flakes)   −1

(e) granola   −2

41. With what do you make tuna salad, pasta salad, chicken salad, etc?

(a) mayonnaise   −2

(b) light mayonnaise   0

(c) low-fat yogurt   +2

(d) nonfat yogurt   +3

42. What do you typically put on your pasta? (Add one point if you also add sautéed vegetables. Average two or more scores if necessary.)

(a) tomato-based sauce   +3

(b) tomato sauce with a little Parmesan   +3

(c) white clam sauce   +1

(d) meat sauce   −1

(e) tomato sauce with meatballs   −2

(f) Alfredo, or other creamy sauce   −3

Total (+)   Total (−)   Your Grand Total

_____ − _____ = _____

+73 TO +127—SUPER!   You're a nutrition superstar. Give yourself a big (nonbutter) pat on the back.

+30 TO +72—GOOD   Pin your quiz to a wall or bulletin
board (with your name in large print,
of course).

−14 TO +29—FAIR   Hang in there. Tape the Center for Science in the Public Interest's Nutrition
Scoreboard poster to your refrigerator
for a little friendly help.

−123 TO −15—ARGHH!   Stop lining the cat box with *Nutrition
Action Healthletter*. Empty your re-
frigerator and cupboard. It's time to
start over.

FAST-FOOD QUIZ

Think you know your fast foods? Let's see.

1. Three of these foods have at least half the fat an average adult
should eat in an entire day. Which one has less?
   (a) McDonald's Biscuit w/Sausage & Egg
   (b) Burger King Whopper w/Cheese
   (c) Domino's Cheese Pizza (2 large slices)
   (d) Arby's Bac'n Cheddar Deluxe
2. Which has the most sodium?
   (a) Arby's Philly Beef 'N Swiss
   (b) Pizza Hut Pepperoni Pan Pizza (2 medium slices)
   (c) Taco Bell Beef Burrito w/red sauce

(d) Hardee's Ham, Egg, & Cheese Biscuit

(e) Kentucky Fried Chicken Extra-Crispy Breast & Thigh

3. Which of these McDonald's foods has the smallest amount of sodium?

(a) Chicken McNuggets

(b) large french fries

(c) chocolate milk shake

(d) chef salad

(e) apple pie

4. Which has more than 1,000 calories?

(a) Dairy Queen Chocolate Malt (large)

(b) Burger King Bacon Double Cheeseburger

(c) Arby's Super Roast Beef Sandwich

(d) Dunkin' Donuts Chocolate Croissant

(e) Wendy's Big Classic

5. Which has as much saturated fat as the average adult should eat in an entire day?

(a) McD.L.T.

(b) Burger King Great Danish

(c) Taco Bell Nachos Bellgrande

(d) Pizza Hut Thin 'n Crispy Medium Supreme Pizza (2 slices)

(e) Hardee's Sausage & Egg Biscuit

6. Which of these McDonald's desserts has the least fat?

(a) Cinnamon Raisin Danish

(b) apple pie

(c) Soft Serve cone

(d) Chocolaty Chip Cookies

■ ANSWERS

1. (c)

2. (e) But all have at least 1,000 mg.

3. (b) You can't tell salt content by taste.

4. (a) But all the others have at least 500 calories.

5. (b) But all the others have at least half that much.

6. (c) All the others have three times as much.

FAST FOODS:
Best and Worst (as of 1989)

Twenty years after America put a man on the moon, three major fast-food restaurants actually began selling nonfried chicken. It's about time.

But the new grilled-chicken sandwiches introduced by Hardee's, Jack-in-the-Box, and Carl's Jr. don't exactly herald the dawning of a new age of healthful fast foods.

The industry leader, McDonald's, for example, has rolled out a fried McChicken Sandwich that has more calories and fat (albeit less saturated fat) than a Quarter Pounder. And Jack-in-the-Box has unveiled the Ultimate Cheeseburger, with enough fat (15¾ teaspoons) to swipe the Coronary Bypass Special title from its previous holder, Wendy's Triple Cheeseburger. Mazel tov.

Fast food is here to stay. One by one, hospitals, colleges, and military installations are caving in to pressure from Ronald McDonald and his cronies. In June a high school in Gilroy, California, actually pleaded with McDonald's, Burger King, and other chains to open a franchise on its campus.

"There's a lot of grease [in the tacos]," a Gilroy senior told *The New York Times*. "But it tastes good, so you don't think about it."

Since fast food is not going to disappear, it's important that the restaurants put some healthful items on their menus, and that consumers have some way to tell the good from the bad.

To that end, we present (in alphabetical order) CSPI's (Center for Science in the Public Interest's) "Best and Worst Fast Foods."

The Worst

Hardee's Big Country Breakfast w/Sausage. If Hardee's Country Breakfast is "big," the heart attacks it may lead to could be "massive."

By your last swallow of scrambled eggs, hash browns, biscuit, and sausages, you will have ingested more than 1,000 calories, 1,950 mg (1 teaspoon) of sodium, a day's worth of cholesterol (280 mg), and more than a day's worth of fat (16 3/4 teaspoons).

We doubt you'll return for lunch.

JACK-IN-THE-BOX ULTIMATE CHEESEBURGER. When Ronald was a McInfant, a hamburger meant just over 1 ounce of cooked ground beef, toppings, and a bun. You can still get a small burger at McDonald's, Burger King, or Wendy's, and size alone makes them some of the best bets on the standard fast-food menu.

But most meat patties (Quarter Pounders and their cousins) now weigh in at 3 ounces after cooking. And extra cheese, bacon, sauces, and/or mayo boost their dose of fat sky-high.

Despite strong competition, Jack-in-the-Box has managed to break the 15½ teaspoon Burger Fat Record previously held by Wendy's Triple Cheeseburger. Along with its 16 teaspoons of fat, Jack's Ultimate packs 942 calories and 1,176 mg of sodium.

ARBY'S ROAST CHICKEN CLUB SANDWICH and McDONALD'S McCHICKEN SANDWICH (tie). Some of the worst fast foods have names that make them sound better than they are. McDonald's new chicken sandwich and Arby's chicken club sandwich are good examples.

Roast chicken sounds innocent enough. Yet Arby's 610-calorie behemoth packs more fat than a Big Mac. The saturated fat content (8 grams) tops Arby's Beef 'N Cheddar sandwich, and the sodium (1,500 mg) beats everything on the menu except the Bac'n Cheddar Deluxe.

It's the cheese, bacon, and mayonnaise that make this sandwich a loser. Either remove them or order something (almost anything) else.

A McChicken Sandwich might seem like a healthful alternative to a burger. But it's fried. All that oil and mayo supply more calories and fat than a Quarter Pounder.

Granted, the fat is less saturated, so it's not as bad for your heart. But your waistline can't tell the difference. Nor is unsaturated fat any better when it comes to raising your risk of breast and colon cancer.

TACO BELL'S TACO LIGHT. It's bad enough that some "light" foods are no lower in fat or calories than their regular counterparts. Now Taco Bell has created a "light" that's actually *worse*.

Your basic unadorned Taco Bell taco (beef, cheese, and lettuce on a tortilla) isn't so bad. It has 183 calories and 2½ teaspoons of fat. Thanks to the sour cream and extra ½ ounce of beef, a Taco Light has more than twice as much of each. That's worse than a Taco Bellgrande, a Soft Taco Supreme, a Super Combo Taco, and a Double Beef Burrito.

A Taco Bell spokesperson told us the taco is called "light" because "it's made with a flour tortilla . . . [which] doesn't absorb as much oil as a corn tortilla when it's fried." Wise up, Taco. The fat's coming from someplace . . . and it isn't the lettuce.

TACO BELL'S TACO SALAD. It's hard to believe, but the fattiest food you can buy at Taco Bell is a salad! With the shell, this platter of beef, cheese, and beans (is that some lettuce hidden under the meat?) packs 14 teaspoons of fat and 941 calories. That's over 90 percent of the fat and 85 percent of the saturated fat the average adult should eat in an entire day.

Even the sodium—all 1,662 mg of it—tops the rest of the Taco Bell menu.

The Winners

Burger King Chicken Salad and *McDonald's Chicken Salad Oriental* (tie). The word "salad" is no guarantee that you're eating light. McDonald's Chef Salad has 3 teaspoons of fat (thanks largely to the egg yolks). That's more than in a hamburger. Even some chicken salads, like Jack-in-the-Box's or Hardee's, are fatty.

That's why McDonald's and Burger King deserve credit for keeping their chicken salads low in fat (under a teaspoon). Burger King's salad, which tasted better to us, has slightly more salt (both chains cook their chicken in a mixture of sodium phosphate, salt, and other seasonings).

The real danger with salads is what you put on them. McDonald's has a tasty, low-fat Oriental dressing, but each tablespoon (there are 4 in a packet) has 180 mg of sodium.

At Burger King, the five salad dressings have anywhere from 115 mg to 215 mg of sodium per tablespoon. And unless you pick the

Reduced-Calorie Italian, each of those tablespoons will add another teaspoon or two of fat to your meal. Use the whole packet, and you end up with as much fat as two hamburgers.

JACK-IN-THE-BOX'S CHICKEN FAJITA PITA. The fast-food fajita is here. A fajita (fah-HEE-tah) consists of grilled strips of chicken or beef and a few vegetables, usually eaten in a rolled-up tortilla.

Jack-in-the-Box's Chicken Fajita Pita is the best so far. It's got slightly less fat (2 teaspoons total) than Taco Bell's chicken or steak fajitas. Even the fattiest fajita (Jack-in-the-Box's beef) isn't fatty by fast-food standards.

If it weren't for the 703 mg of sodium, the Chicken Fajita would be close to perfect. Change your seasoning, Jack!

TACO BELL BEAN BURRITO. Although the chef adds corn oil to the beans, the finished burrito has only about 2 teaspoons of fat and a mere 9 mg of cholesterol. Not bad.

Sodium is on the high side (763 mg with green sauce, 888 mg with red sauce), but it's still below the beef burritos and taco salads.

Honorable Mentions

Carl's Jr. Charbroiler BBQ Chicken Sandwich. This smallish West Coast chain specializes in fat-laden burgers, but its charbroiled chicken sandwich rates an Honorable Mention.

The BBQ's single teaspoon of fat contributes only 14 percent of its calories. Low-fat barbecue sauce in place of mayo means the Charbroiler is even leaner than Hardee's Grilled Chicken Sandwich. But sodium is still excessive at 955 mg. On the plus side, you get a honey-wheat (not to be confused with 100 percent whole wheat) bun.

HARDEE'S GRILLED CHICKEN SANDWICH. Hardee's is certainly trying. Though its menu is splattered with disasters like the Big Country Breakfast, the chain is one of the few in the burger business to cook its french fries in vegetable oil rather than beef tallow.

Now Hardee's gets an Honorable Mention for its tasty Grilled

Chicken Sandwich, which has less than 3 teaspoons of fat. That's almost one third less than Jack-in-the-Box's Grilled Chicken Fillet and less than half what you'd get in a McDonald's (fried) McChicken Sandwich.

If you ask Hardee's to hold the (reduced-calorie) mayo, you get only about 1 teaspoon of fat. Like Carl's Jr., you get a multigrain bun. It too is less than 100 percent whole wheat, but considering the cotton-puff buns most fast-food sandwiches are served on, it's a milestone.

If it weren't for the Grilled Chicken Sandwich's 1,240 mg of sodium, Hardee's would have a winner.

THE BEST, THE WORST, AND (SOME OF THE) REST

	Calories	Fat (tsp)[1]	Sodium (mg)[2]	Gloom[3]
BREAKFAST FOODS				
McDONALD'S English Muffin w/butter	169	1	270	9
McDONALD'S Hotcakes w/Butter & Syrup	413	2	640	20
McDONALD'S Egg McMuffin	293	2¾	740	25
McDONALD'S Biscuit w/Sausage & Egg	529	8	1,250	57
BURGER KING Croissanwich w/Sausage	538	9¼	1,042	61*
W HARDEE'S Big Country Breakfast (Sausage)	1,005	16¾	1,950	97
BURGERS				
McDONALD'S Hamburger	257	2¼	460	17
McDONALD'S Quarter Pounder w/ Cheese	517	6¾	1,150	45
WENDY'S Big Classic w/Cheese	640	9	1,310	56*
McDONALD'S McD.L.T.	674	9½	1,170	56
WENDY'S Triple Cheeseburger	1,040	15½	1,848	85*
W JACK-IN-THE-BOX Ultimate Cheeseburger	942	15¾	1,176	88
CHICKEN SANDWICHES				
B CARL'S JR. BBQ Chicken Sandwich	320	1¼	955	17
B HARDEE's Grilled Chicken Sandwich	330	2¾	1,240	25

		Calories	Fat (tsp)[1]	Sodium (mg)[2]	Gloom[3]
	JACK-IN-THE-BOX Grilled Chicken Fillet Sandwich	408	3¾	1,130	29
	WENDY'S Chicken Breast Fillet Sandwich	430	4¼	705	27*
	ARBY'S Chicken Breast Sandwich	493	5¾	1,019	33
W	McDONALD'S McChicken Sandwich	490	6½	780	39
W	ARBY'S Roast Chicken Club Sandwich	610	8½	1,500	53

MEXICAN FOODS

B	JACK-IN-THE-BOX Chicken Fajita Pita	292	1¾	703	16
	TACO BELL Chicken Fajita	226	2¼	619	18*
B	TACO BELL Bean Burrito w/Green Sauce	351	2¼	763	17*
	TACO BELL Taco	183	2½	276	16*
	TACO BELL Steak Fajita	234	2½	485	18*
	JACK-IN-THE-BOX Beef Fajita Pita	333	3¼	635	22
	TACO BELL Super Combo Taco	286	3½	462	23*
W	TACO BELL Taco Light	410	6½	594	39*

SALADS (NO DRESSINGS ADDED)

B	McDONALD'S Chicken Salad Oriental	141	¾	230	7
B	BURGER KING Chicken Salad	140	1	440	9
	McDONALD'S Chef Salad	231	3	490	21
	HARDEE's Chicken Fiesta Salad	286	3¼	533	26
	JACK-IN-THE-BOX Mexican Chicken Salad	442	5¼	1,500	41
	TACO BELL Taco Salad w/out Shell	520	7	1,431	47*
	WENDY'S Taco Salad	660	8½	1,110	45*
W	TACO BELL Taco Salad w/Shell	941	14	1,662	75*

All information obtained from manufacturers.
[1] To convert teaspoons of fat to grams, multiply by 4.4.
[2] The recommended daily sodium intake for an adult is 2,400 mg.
[3] Center for Science in the Public Interest's "Gloom" rating ranks food according to their fat, sodium, cholesterol, and vitamin and mineral content. The higher the number, the worse the food.
*"Gloom" rating was estimated without full information on fat content from manufacturer.

TEST YOUR OVERALL NUTRITION KNOWLEDGE

It seems as if everyone is talking or writing about nutrition these days. Even if you seldom follow the subject, you might be surprised at the amount of information you have absorbed subliminally. A form of mind control, some might say.

1. How many grams of fiber do nutritionists recommend that adults consume each day?
   (a) 5 to 10
   (b) 10 to 15
   (c) 20 to 35
   (d) 50 to 75
2. Which fruit contains the most fiber?
   (a) prunes
   (b) dried figs
   (c) pears
   (d) bananas
   (e) raspberries
3. When orange juice is pasteurized, how much of its vitamin C does it lose?
   (a) no more than 5 percent
   (b) 10–15 percent
   (c) 50 percent
   (d) almost all
4. Olestra is
   (a) a recently discovered form of good cholesterol
   (b) an artificial sugar
   (c) an edible form of polyester
   (d) an artificial fat
5. As long as food contains no cholesterol, anyone on a low-cholesterol diet can eat it. True or false?
6. How does wheat bread differ from white bread?
   (a) it has whole-wheat flour in it
   (b) it is made with 100 percent whole wheat flour
   (c) it is no different from white bread
7. Many people, especially women, have been taking calcium supplements in recent years to help prevent osteoporosis, a crippling bone disease that is related to a calcium deficiency. True or false:
   (a) All bone formation stops once you reach adulthood.

   (b) Calcium is used for other functions in the body besides build-
       ing bones and teeth.

   (c) Taking calcium supplements is the best way to prevent
       osteoporosis.

8. The word "light" or "lite" on a label means

   (a) The product is lighter in color than the standard version.

   (b) The product has fewer calories than the standard version.

   (c) The product has less sodium than the standard version.

   (d) The product has less fat than the standard version.

   (e) Any of the above.

9. While sweeteners are seldom listed first in the ingredient statement on food packaging, some packaged foods contain more
sweeteners than any other ingredient. True or false?

■ **ANSWERS**

1. The correct answer is 20 to 35 grams, nutrition experts say.

   Most Americans probably consume far less. There can also be
too much of a good thing: 50 to 75 grams a day can cause intestinal problems and can allow certain minerals like zinc to leach out
of the body.

2. The answer is prunes.

   According to the Department of Agriculture's Handbook 8,
which lists nutritional values of foods, prunes have 2.04 grams of
dietary fiber per 100 grams.

3. The answer is 10 to 15 percent, according to tests done by the
government and the food industry.

   Most commercially available orange juice is pasteurized, a process in which the juice is heated to 195 degrees for 10 to 15 seconds
to kill harmful bacteria and prolong its shelf life. In that short
period of time not much vitamin C is destroyed. A 6-ounce glass of
pasteurized orange juice will yield 70 mg of vitamin C, which is 120
percent of the U.S. Recommended Daily Allowance.

4. Olestra is an artificial fat produced by the Procter & Gamble Co.

   Because the compound passes through the body without being
digested, it adds no calories or cholesterol. But the Food and
Drug Administration has not yet approved its use in food for

humans; the company's safety studies are still under scrutiny by the agency.

5. False.

Eating too much dietary cholesterol is not the only way to raise blood cholesterol levels.

Too much saturated fat will have the same effect. Anyone on a low-cholesterol diet must reduce the intake of products containing animal fats as well as saturated fats like coconut oil, palm oil, and palm kernel oil. While dietary cholesterol and saturated fat are not the same thing, both raise blood-cholesterol levels. Even though a product may say "no cholesterol" on the label, if it contains saturated fat, it is not good for anyone on a low-cholesterol diet.

6. Wheat bread is the same as white bread.

It contains no whole wheat flour, and if it is a different color from white bread, the color probably comes from caramel coloring. Bread labeled "100 percent whole wheat," however, must be made with whole wheat flour, and therefore contains more fiber.

7. (a) False.

Bone formation and reformation go on continuously.

(b) True.

Calcium also helps your heart to beat, your muscles to work, your blood to clot, and your nerves to function.

(c) False.

Taking calcium may prevent further progression of osteoporosis, but there are many other factors involved in preventing the disease: regular exercise, cessation of smoking, and reduced stress.

8. Any of the above.

There are no government standards regulating terms for such products.

9. True.

The ingredients on food packaging are listed in order of predominance, but some products contain sweeteners in several forms. This is particularly true in cereals, where corn syrup, brown sugar, and dextrose may all be added. Singly they are not the predominant ingredient; collectively they are.

ARE YOU UP ON YOUR FACTS ABOUT FAT?

Are you aware of hidden fats in the foods you eat? Do you know that some fats can increase your risk of a stroke or a heart attack, while other fats can lower those risks? Take this quiz to see how much you really know about fat and nutrition. You won't need a pencil, just your wits. And put away those potato chips. They're fried in oil.

1. First things first. Do we or don't we *need* fats in our diet?
   Yes, we do   Go to 7
   No, we don't   Go to 10

2. Bad show. There are just over 4 calories per gram (about the weight of two paper clips) in both carbohydrates and proteins, but 9 in fats. Try 4 again.

3. Which of the following has the highest amount of fat?
   4 ounces of tofu   Go to 6
   1 medium avocado   Go to 9
   8 ounces of chili   Go to 12

4. Is that chocolate ice cream you're eating? There are about 7 grams of fat in a ½ cup scoop. Each gram of fat has how many calories?
   4   Go to 2
   9   Go to 8
   18   Go to 11

5. Of course there's more to it than just calories. Do fats raise your blood-cholesterol level?
   Yes   Go to 21
   No   Go to 13

6. Nope.

   Four ounces of tofu have 5 grams of fat. By the way, if you don't know what tofu is made of, read 17. If you do know, try 3 again.

7. Good start.

   Fats provide essential nutrients. They are a source of linoleic acid and vitamins A, D, E, and K. Go to 4 now and a question about the calories in the fats we eat.

8. There you go.

   Every gram of fat contains 9 calories, no matter what form it's in. Whether it's ice cream or steak, fat is fat. Try 3 now.

9. Yes, that's right.

   Avocados are *packed* with fat. One medium avocado has 32 grams! Eat fewer avocados, perhaps? Now to 14.

10. Ah, too bad.

    We *do* need fats in our diet, though not nearly as much as most of us get. Why don't you go back to 1 and pretend you're just beginning?

11. Ooh, you're way off.

    Try 4 again.

12. Sorry.

    One cup of chili has about 11 grams of fat. Try 3 again.

13. Yes and no.

    To learn why, go to 21.

14. And how about these foods? Which of the following are generally lowest in fat?

    Cheeses   Go to 19
    Grains   Go to 20
    Nuts   Go to 24

15. Sure.

    Saturated fats are mostly derived from animals and are usually solid at room temperature. But watch out for two vegetable oils: coconut and palm oils. Both are saturated fats. To 28 now, comin' down the stretch.

16. Yes and no.

Polyunsaturated fats come in two major forms: the omega-6 fatty acids that are in almost all vegetable oils and the omega-3s, found predominantly in cold-water fish such as salmon and mackerel. Studies suggest that both types help reduce cholesterol and body weight. And omega-3s in fish also appear to reduce bad (LDL) cholesterol levels. So you might want to substitute fish for at least two red-meat meals each week. Now read 23.

17. Tofu, a popular health food, is simply soybean curds, rich in protein and high in polyunsaturated fat. Back to 3 now.

18. Saturated fats include
Beef fat, butter, lard   Go to 15
Fatty fish, soy oil, olive oil Go to 26

19. Wrong.

Nearly all cheese is high in fat. In fact, a number of popular cheeses, including cheddar and Roquefort, are over 70 percent fat. Back to 14 for another try.

20. Good choice.

Almost all grain products are under 30 percent fat. Beware of those processed in oil. Otherwise you're on pretty safe ground. Proceed to 5.

21. Well, you're right and you're wrong.

Most saturated fats do raise cholesterol levels and should be avoided, while many unsaturated fats actually help reverse the trend. Move on to 18.

22. Yikes! Pretty strict, aren't you?

Unless you're on a special low-cholesterol diet, all fats should be reduced to less than 30 percent, with saturated fats lowered by at least 10 percent. Go back to 29 and don't be so hard on yourself.

23. Attaway. But don't be so smug.

Monounsaturated fats (most commonly consumed today in olive and peanut oils) are thought to reduce those bad (LDL) cholesterol levels. Go back to 16 before you proceed to 29 and a final question.

24. Guess again.

Nuts, as well as products made from nuts—peanut butter, for example—are very high in fat. To keep within the less than 30 percent guideline, eat peanut butter in moderation.

25. That's the one.

For those with high cholesterol levels, no more than 10 percent is recommended. Now to 30 for a wrap-up.

26. Aw, c'mon. You can do better than that.

In general, animal fats are saturated (unhealthful) and vegetable oils are unsaturated (healthful). Notable exceptions are palm oil and coconut oil, which are saturated fats, and fish, which is unsaturated fat. Go to 28 and bear down a bit more.

27. Fifty-three percent. Bye.

28. And of the unsaturated fats, which are better for you?
Polyunsaturated   Go to 16
Monounsaturated   Go to 23

29. Okay, so you're convinced. You should lower your overall fat intake and stay away from most saturated fats. According to the American Heart Association and the National Institutes of Health, what percentage of your daily caloric intake can be from fat?
8 percent   Go to 22
30 percent   Go to 25

30. Done! How you did doesn't matter as long as you enjoyed yourself and learned a few things along the way. Before you go, can you guess what percentage of the calories in a McDonald's Big Mac come from saturated fat? See 27 for the answer.

ARE YOU AT RISK OF OBESITY?

Nearly one in ten Americans is 30 percent above his or her desirable body weight and, therefore, at a greater health risk than those of normal weight. So says Steven B. Heymsfield, M.D.—and he should know, for he's the director of outpatient obesity and human body composition core units of the Obesity Research Center at St. Luke's-Roosevelt Hospital Center in New York. His observations echo the findings of the National Institutes of Health, whose 1987 conference on the topic detailed these health risks of obesity: diabe-

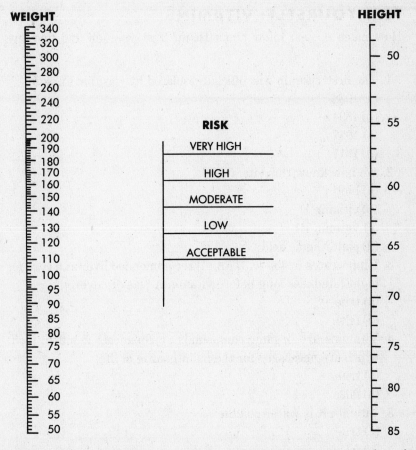

Weight is in pounds, height in inches. Place a straight edge across height and weight, and read health risk of obesity on the vertical line.

tes, heart disease, high blood pressure, certain types of cancer, and other chronic, disabling conditions.

Are you at risk of obesity? The necessary first step—certainly before selecting and embarking on an appropriate weight-loss program—is to answer that question. To that end, Dr. Heymsfield has designed a chart (see page 57), that will help you determine whether you are above your desirable body weight.

TEST YOURSELF: VITAMINS

How much do you know about them? Test yourself and find out.

1. The first vitamin was officially isolated by Casimir Funk in
   (a) 1938
   (b) 1894
   (c) 1977
   (d) 1911
2. We now know this vitamin as
   (a) biotin
   (b) vitamin D
   (c) vitamin B1
   (d) pantothenic acid
3. Hippocrates (c.460–c.377 B.C.) recommended liver as a cure for night blindness long before vitamin A was discovered:
   (a) true
   (b) false
4. Vitamins are organic compounds or chemicals found in food, which are necessary for the maintenance of life:
   (a) true
   (b) false
5. Vitamin K is water-soluble:
   (a) true
   (b) false
6. Vitamin B3 is also known as

(a) niacin
(b) niacinamide
(c) nicotinic acid
(d) nicotinamide
(e) all of the above

7. The fat-soluble vitamins contain carbon, hydrogen, and oxygen, and the water-soluble vitamins contain these three elements as well as
(a) plutonium
(b) aspartic acid
(c) nitrogen
(d) helium

8. Vitamin A can be taken in unlimited amounts without any problems:
(a) true
(b) false

9. If you are deficient in vitamin C, your body simply produces more:
(a) true
(b) false

10. In addition to food sources such as fish oils, vitamin D is available from
(a) intestinal flora
(b) bottled water
(c) limestone
(d) sunshine

11. Adermin was the original name for
(a) vitamin C
(b) baldness
(c) vitamin A
(d) vitamin B6

12. Which vitamin has been used successfully to treat arthritis?
(a) vitamin B3
(b) vitamin A
(c) vitamin E
(d) lecithin

13. Choline, inositol, and para-amino benzoic acid are officially B vitamins:
    (a) true
    (b) false

14. The new Recommended Dietary Allowances include which of the following for the first time?
    (a) zinc and vitamin D
    (b) nitrogen and echinacea
    (c) vitamin K and selenium
    (d) carnitine and vitamin E

15. The Recommended Dietary Allowances are published about every five years by a government agency:
    (a) true
    (b) false

16. Researchers have reported encouraging results using niacin to treat
    (a) blood clots
    (b) cancer
    (c) thalassemia
    (d) insomnia

17. When you see a reference to vitamin H, it means:
    (a) hesperidin
    (b) histidine
    (c) biotin
    (d) vitamin B2

18. The bottles on the shelf of the health food store read "panto-thenic acid," but researchers sometimes call it:
    (a) Williams acid
    (b) vitamin B5
    (c) pangamic acid
    (d) pau d'arco

■ ANSWERS

1. (d) 1911

2. (c) vitamin B1 (thiamine)

3. (a) true.

He did not know at the time what substance in the liver was responsible.

4. (a) true.

They are also available in concentrated form as food supplements.

5. (b) false.

It's fat-soluble, which means that it is stored in body fat.

6. (e) All of the above

7. (c) Nitrogen

8. (b) false.

Safe amounts for adults generally are in the 10,000 to 25,000 IU range. Toxic reactions can occur with excessive dosage.

9. (b) false

10. (d) sunshine

11. (d) vitamin B6

12. (a) vitamin B3

13. (b) false.

They are water-soluble substances that are part of the B complex vitamins but are not actually B vitamins.

14. (c) vitamin K and selenium

15. (b) false.

They are issued by the National Research Council, which is a nonprofit organization.

16. (b) cancer

17. (c) biotin (a member of the B complex vitamins found in all living tissue)

18. (b) vitamin B5

■ SCORING

A score of 16–18 is excellent; 13–15 is good; 11–12 is fair; 10 or below means you need to study more!

DO YOU KNOW WHERE THE SODIUM IS IN YOUR DIET?

Over the past few decades, the subject of salt in the diet has grown into a full-blown health issue. The mineral sodium—a part of many foods and food additives—is necessary for human well-being. Salt, which is 40 percent sodium, is the vehicle by which most of us get our daily portion of sodium. The problem is—our daily portion is just too high. Most of us are sopping up as much as *30 times* the amount our bodies actually *need*. And while most of us don't have any adverse reaction to sodium, it's likely that a large minority percentage of people are genetically programmed to react to sodium by a rise in blood pressure.

What to do? A concerned person will be careful not to overdo and will eat smart. The general medical advice to the person with high blood pressure is to go on a low-salt diet and, perhaps along with anti-hypertensive drugs and other therapies, see whether that helps. The person with normal blood pressure should control the urge to salt everything—just in case.

Keeping the salt shaker off your table is easy, but how can you restrict the sodium in your diet *if you don't know where it is?* First things first: The Food and Drug Administration says that, aside from table salt, at least 70 other sodium compounds are being used in foods today. Here's a quiz to test whether you have even a grain of understanding about some of the more common sodium compounds (many of these should be very familiar to you if you read the labels on your food). Match the compound and its use.

1. sodium chloride
2. monosodium glutamate
3. sodium bicarbonate
4. baking powder
5. disodium phosphate
6. sodium alginate
7. sodium benzoate
8. sodium hydroxide
9. sodium nitrite
10. sodium propionate
11. sodium sulfite

(a) Used in many chocolate milks and ice creams to make the mixture smooth

(b) Used to leaven breads and cakes; added to vegetables during cooking; used as an alkalizer for indigestion; also called baking soda

(c) Used as a preservative in some dried fruits such as prunes; used to bleach certain fruits such as glazed or crystallized ones that are to be artificially colored

(d) Used in pasteurized cheese and in some breads and cakes to inhibit mold growth

(e) Used in cooking or at the table; used in canning and preserving

(f) Present in some quick-cooking cereals and processed cheeses

(g) Used in food processing to soften and loosen skins of ripe olives and some fruits and vegetables

(h) Used in home, restaurant, and hotel cooking, and in many packaged, canned, and frozen foods

(i) Used as a preservative in many condiments such as relishes, sauces, and salad dressings

(j) Used in cured meats and sausages

(k) Used to leaven quick breads, cakes, and biscuits

■ **ANSWERS**

1—(e)	7—(i)
2—(h)	8—(g)
3—(b)	9—(j)
4—(k)	10—(d)
5—(f)	11—(c)
6—(a)	

The American Heart Association recommends that you limit your intake of items 1 through 4. Good advice—but also don't forget, as this quiz amply illustrates, to watch for the "hidden" sodium in canned, frozen, or otherwise processed foods. Canned vegetables often have salt added to them. Even canned fruits may have salt in them. Certain antacids are high in sodium, and even *naturally occurring* sodium can slip into your tummy unbeknownst to the most scrupulous dietitians. One of the sneakiest is milk, although celery, artichokes, and spinach have moderate amounts, too. And some drinking water may have a lot of natural sodium in it.

HOW LOW DO YOU GO? DO YOU KNOW?

Understanding the language of low-salt is not easy. That's because when food manufacturers and packagers speak of the amount of sodium in a product, they speak in terms of grams and milligrams. A gram—usually abbreviated *g* on labels—is a unit of weight, but, unless you are a research chemist or have voluntarily converted to the metric system in your household, you probably have no idea what this translates to in the real world. Here's a quick lesson: There are approximately 28 grams in 1 ounce, and there are 5.5 grams in a teaspoon. And 1,000 milligrams (mg) equal 1 gram.

According to the American Heart Association, the average American consumes about 6 to 18 grams of salt daily—that's about 1 to 2 teaspoonfuls—even though the National Academy of Sciences says that daily sodium consumption of from 1,100 to 3,300 milligrams (1.1 to 3.3 grams) is a safe and adequate amount. As you can see, Americans consume far more than that.

Part of the problem no doubt lies in consumer misunderstanding or outright ignorance of sodium levels in various products. Health concerns about sodium (along with eagerness to turn a profit on the growing market demand for healthy food) have prompted quite a number of manufacturers to describe their products as low in sodium. These claims are often made on food product labels. (Watch for the words *sodium* or *soda*, and the symbol *Na*—they all identify products containing sodium compounds.) In order to ensure uniformity in their use by manufacturers and thus avoid consumer confusion, the Food and Drug Administration (FDA) has provided a set of descriptive terms to use for the claims.

In this quiz, see if you can match the FDA-specified terms with the descriptions. If you can't, there's a good chance you're consuming more sodium than you intend to and/or that is recommended:

1. Sodium free

    (a) 35 mg or less sodium per serving

2. Very low sodium

    (b) Foods for which the usual level of sodium has been cut by at least 75 percent

3. Moderately low sodium

    (c) 140 mg or less sodium per serving

4. Reduced sodium

    (d) Food once processed with salt but now produced without it—however, may contain other forms of sodium

5. Unsalted, or no salt added, or some equivalent

    (e) Less than 5 mg of sodium per serving

■ **ANSWERS**

1—(e)   4—(b)
2—(a)   5—(d)
3—(c)

TESTING YOUR SODIUM SAVVY

That was easy, right? Now, let's see whether you truly are in the know about no-, low-, and high-sodium foods. Of the two choices given, circle the one you believe is *lower* in sodium. (Assume nearly equal weight or portion, and consider neither to contain added table salt or to be specially designated low-salt.) Then check the answers below for the comparative milligrams of sodium.

1. (a) tomato juice
   (b) grapefruit juice

2. (a) Wheaties cereal
   (b) Sugar Corn Pops cereal

3. (a) Rice Krispies cereal
   (b) Trix cereal

4. (a) Instant Cream of Wheat
   (b) Quick Cream of Wheat

5. (a) 1 frozen cinnamon Danish
   (b) 1 yeast-leavened doughnut

6. (a) 1 frozen cinnamon sweet roll
   (b) 1 frosted cinnamon toaster pastry

7. (a) Cheddar cheese
   (b) blue cheese

8. (a) ricotta (whole-milk)
   (b) cottage cheese (regular or low-fat)

9. (a) American cheese
   (b) Colby cheese

10. (a) whole or low-fat milk
    (b) instantized dry nonfat milk

11. (a) frankfurter
    (b) canned light tuna (water-packed)

12. (a) olive loaf
    (b) turkey roll

13. (a) chicken spread
    (b) deviled ham

14. (a) mixed grain bread
    (b) refrigerated dough roll

15. (a) saltine cracker
    (b) twist pretzel

16. (a) caramel popcorn
    (b) regular popcorn (salt and oil)

17. (a) roasted, salted almonds
    (b) dry-roasted, salted peanuts

18. (a) frozen meat loaf dinner
    (b) frozen Swiss steak dinner

19. (a) frozen tuna pot pie
    (b) frozen turkey pot pie

20. (a) veal parmigiana
    (b) canned ravioli

21. (a) frozen shrimp dinner
    (b) canned sweet and sour pork

22. (a) canned green peas
    (b) raw broccoli

23. (a) cooked beets
    (b) canned sliced beets

24. (a) canned lima beans
    (b) frozen lima beans

25. (a) mashed potatoes (with milk and salt)
    (b) potatoes au gratin

26. (a) potato salad
    (b) cole slaw

27. (a) canned kidney beans
    (b) canned Boston-style baked beans

28. (a) condensed (reconstituted with water) chicken noodle soup
    (b) condensed (reconstituted with water) chicken rice soup

29. (a) condensed (reconstituted with water) Manhattan clam chowder
    (b) condensed (reconstituted with water) tomato soup

30. (a) sugar cookie
    (b) 6 vanilla wafer cookies

31. (a) frozen chocolate Bavarian cream pie
    (b) frozen mince pie

32. (a) devil's food cake
    (b) angel food cake

33. (a) licorice candy
    (b) peanut brittle

34. (a) milk chocolate candy
    (b) taffy

35. (a) brown sugar
    (b) granulated sugar

■ ANSWERS

1. (a) tomato juice, 878 mg
   (b) grapefruit juice, 4 mg

2. (a) Wheaties cereal, 355 mg
   (b) Sugar Corn Pops cereal, 105 mg

3. (a) Rice Krispies cereal, 340 mg
   (b) Trix cereal, 160 mg

4. (a) Instant Cream of Wheat, 5 mg
   (b) Quick Cream of Wheat, 126 mg

5. (a) 1 frozen cinnamon Danish, 260 mg
   (b) 1 yeast-leavened doughnut, 99 mg

6. (a) 1 frozen cinnamon sweet roll, 110 mg
   (b) 1 frosted cinnamon toaster pastry, 326 mg

7. (a) Cheddar cheese, 176 mg
   (b) blue cheese, 396 mg

8. (a) ricotta (whole-milk), 104 mg
   (b) cottage cheese (regular or low-fat), 457 mg

9. (a) American cheese, 406 mg
   (b) Colby cheese, 171 mg

10. (a) whole or low-fat milk, 122 mg
    (b) instantized dry nonfat milk, 373 mg

11. (a) frankfurter, 639 mg
    (b) canned light tuna (water-packed), 288 mg

12. (a) olive loaf, 312 mg
    (b) turkey roll, 166 mg

13. (a) chicken spread, 115 mg
    (b) deviled ham, 253 mg

14. (a) mixed grain bread, 138 mg
    (b) refrigerated dough roll, 342 mg

15. (a) saltine cracker, 35 mg
    (b) twist pretzel, 101 mg

16. (a) caramel popcorn, 262 mg
    (b) regular popcorn (salt and oil), 175 mg

17. (a) roasted, salted almonds, 311 mg
    (b) dry-roasted, salted peanuts, 986 mg

18. (a) frozen meat loaf dinner, 1,304 mg
    (b) frozen Swiss steak dinner, 682 mg

19. (a) frozen tuna pot pie, 715 mg
    (b) frozen turkey pot pie, 1,018 mg

20. (a) veal parmigiana, 1,825 mg
    (b) canned ravioli, 1,065 mg

21. (a) frozen shrimp dinner, 758 mg
    (b) canned sweet and sour pork, 1,968 mg

22. (a) canned green peas, 493 mg
    (b) raw broccoli, 23 mg

23. (a) cooked beets, 73 mg
    (b) canned sliced beets, 479 mg

24. (a) canned lima beans, 456 mg
    (b) frozen lima beans, 128 mg

25. (a) mashed potatoes (with milk and salt), 632 mg
    (b) potatoes au gratin, 1,095 mg

26. (a) potato salad, 625 mg
    (b) cole slaw, 68 mg

27. (a) canned kidney beans, 844 mg
    (b) canned Boston-style baked beans, 606 mg

28. (a) condensed chicken noodle soup, 1,107 mg
    (b) condensed chicken rice soup, 814 mg

29. (a) condensed Manhattan clam chowder, 1,029 mg
    (b) condensed tomato soup, 872 mg

30. (a) sugar cookie, 108 mg
    (b) 6 vanilla wafer cookies, 53 mg

31. (a) frozen chocolate Bavarian cream pie (⅛ pie), 78 mg
    (b) frozen mince pie (⅛ pie), 258 mg

32. (a) devil's food cake (¹⁄₁₂ cake), 402 mg
    (b) angel food cake (¹⁄₁₂ cake), 134 mg

33. (a) licorice candy, 28 mg
    (b) peanut brittle, 145 mg

34. (a) milk chocolate candy, 28 mg
    (b) taffy, 88 mg

35. (a) brown sugar, 66 mg
    (b) granulated sugar, 2 mg

3. CHECK YOURSELF OUT

Eighty-five percent of all medical care in this country is self-care. Consumers diagnose everything from sore throats to knee bruises, and prescribe treatments for themselves in far greater numbers than doctors. Much of what we call self-care is old home remedies: lotions and potions that have passed from generation to generation. Most often they work for the minor ailments we all encounter. Sometimes they work for more complex, serious conditions.

Self-care and self-diagnosis are growing by leaps and bounds in this country. Much of what we always held as strictly within a physician's domain is now available to the public. The last section of this book describes twenty-one tests that you can do at home. Until just a few years ago each one required a visit to either a doctor's office or a hospital. Indeed, things are changing.

But there are other tests doctors use that require no fancy or complicated medical instruments. These are tests that require observation, the honest answering of some questions, and, in some cases, a few simple instructions. We have put twelve of those tests together in this chapter.

We call this chapter "Check Yourself Out" because, to a certain extent, every test allows you to be your own doctor. The tests give you the opportunity to be a major and active participant in your own diagnostics and care. And, of course, if one or more of these tests suggest you might have a problem, you should seek further professional consultation.

TEST YOUR HEALTH IQ

Think you've got a healthy knowledge of health, diet, and fitness? Then take this test. Get ten or more right, and you're using your head for a healthier body.

1. Which of these is *not* a factor in causing high blood pressure (over 140/90), which affects up to one of every four Americans?
   (a) stress
   (b) age
   (c) changes in air pressure
   (d) physical condition
   (e) genetics

2. The average American feels bad enough either to take the day off from work or restrict physical activity due to sniffling, coughing, colds, flus, or other ailments on how many days each year, according to the National Center for Health Statistics?
   (a) 3 days
   (b) 6 days
   (c) 10 days
   (d) 14 days

3. What impact does a full moon reportedly have on a woman's sex drive?
   (a) It increases it by about 30 percent.
   (b) It decreases it by about 10 percent.
   (c) It has no effect.

4. Which of the following is not in the legume family?
   (a) pinto beans

(b) string beans

(c) peas

(d) All are legumes.

5. When looking for a good walking shoe, look for all of the following *except*

(a) breathable construction material such as leather or canvas

(b) a somewhat pointed toe box to help keep feet snug during long walks

(c) a stiff heel counter to support the heel and prevent the foot from leaning

6. Not taking metabolism or the type of foods eaten into account, those trying to lose weight through dieting and daily exercise can generally eat how much more food than those on a diet-only reduction program and still lose weight?

(a) None, but exercise lessens the amount of muscle tissue lost by eating fewer calories.

(b) 10 percent more

(c) 25 percent more

(d) As much as he or she wants; dieting is not needed if you exercise regularly

7. Which activity burns the most calories in an hour?

(a) walking

(b) swimming

(c) rowing

(d) bicycling

8. Which is most likely to cause food-related illness because of carried toxins, bacteria, and viruses, according to former FDA Commissioner Frank Young?

(a) chicken

(b) fish

(c) beef

(d) produce sprayed by Alar

9. Generally, the darker a vegetable's color, the more nutrients it contains.

(a) true

(b) false

10. Vegetables boiled in water retain more vitamins and minerals than those cooked in a microwave oven.
    (a) true
    (b) false

11. Long-term sun exposure can increase your risk of developing cataracts by how much?
    (a) 10 percent
    (b) doubles the risk
    (c) triples the risk

12. If you have heartburn, which of the following should you *not* do:
    (a) sleep on an incline by placing blocks of wood under the headposts of your bed
    (b) lose excess weight
    (c) consume chocolate, peppermint, or spearmint
    (d) wear loose-fitting belts

13. Anything above this cholesterol reading puts you at borderline risk:
    (a) 180
    (b) 200
    (c) 240
    (d) 300

14. Which of the following cooking oils has the highest percentage of saturated fats?
    (a) safflower oil
    (b) olive oil
    (c) coconut oil
    (d) corn oil

15. Which is lowest in saturated fats?
    (a) safflower oil
    (b) olive oil
    (c) coconut oil
    (d) corn oil

■ **ANSWERS**

1. (c)	9. (a)
2. (d)	10. (b)
3. (a)	11. (c)
4. (d)	12. (c)
5. (b)	13. (b)
6. (c)	14. (c)
7. (c)	15. (a)
8. (b)	

HOW FIT ARE YOU?

If a last-minute dash through the airport sets your heart tap dancing in your chest or if lifting a bag of groceries strains your back, you've experienced one of the best motivators for shaping up.

"When everyday activities make you huff and puff," says Stanford University's Abby King, "you know you're not as fit as you want to be."

But just how fit—or unfit—are you? Tests that assess your fitness level and let you compare yourself with norms for your age and sex can be a good way to find out.

"Fitness tests help you set up a baseline to compare yourself with, six weeks or six months from now," says King, who helps direct a Stanford program geared to encouraging adults to be more active. When—after exercising regularly—you discover that a sprint around the block takes you four minutes instead of six, King says, "That's a real motivator."

"It's not until some sort of accounting is made that people will make a conscious effort to change," says Tony Evans, director of exercise science at Pacific Lutheran University in Tacoma, Washington. That accounting may come from a physical examination, which is recommended before beginning an exercise program for sedentary individuals, people over 45, or those of any age with risk factors of heart disease. Or, for otherwise healthy individuals, it can come from tests you give yourself that help you keep track of your progress as you exercise.

One of the easiest fitness tests you can give yourself is to take your pulse. "Your pulse gives you very good feedback about how hard you're working and what shape you're in," King says.

To take your pulse, locate your carotid artery, which starts at the base of the throat and runs vertically up the front of your neck and then behind your ear. Or find the artery at the inside of your wrist, and press your fingers on it, just below your thumb. Count the number of times your heart beats in 10 seconds. Multiply that by 6 to find out the number of beats per minute.

"You can do something simple like walk up and down the stairs for one minute, keeping a standard pace in your head," King says. "Then take your pulse. Take the same test again, after a month or two of a regular fitness program. You should see a drop in your pulse rate, because as you get more fit, your body has gotten more efficient at doing the same amount of work."

For more complete assessments, you should consider four areas, says Robert McMurray, director of the exercise physiology lab at the University of North Carolina at Chapel Hill. These include the following:

■ AEROBIC FITNESS. "This test determines the capacity of the heart to pump blood to the muscles," McMurray says. Several running or walking tests have been developed for individual use. One of the newest is the Rockport Fitness Walking Test, which is based on the time it takes you to walk one mile.

"The more fit you are, the more oxygen you are capable of utilizing," says Ann Wade, an exercise physiologist at the University of Massachusetts Medical School and one of the developers of the test. "Our studies show that you can get an accurate estimation of an individual's aerobic capacity from age, body weight, gender, the time it takes to walk one mile, and the heart-rate response to the one-mile walk."

■ FLEXIBILITY. "Determining your range of motion is particularly important if you will be working in a sport," says McMurray. "If your muscles are too tight or too loose, it can increase the probability of injury."

McMurray recommends two flexibility tests. One is a "sit and reach" test, done sitting on the floor with legs extended in front to gauge flexibility of the hamstring muscle group in the back of the legs. "If you can lean forward and touch your toes without bending your knees, you have good flexibility," he says. This test is important for people with low back pain, which is associated with tightness in those muscles.

The other test is for flexibility in the shoulder area. Reach one arm up and back and the other arm down and back, trying to shake hands with yourself behind your back. "If you can get your thumbs within two inches of each other," he says, "that's pretty good."

■ MUSCLE STRENGTH. The number of sit-ups and push-ups you can do in one minute offers an assessment of muscle strength, McMurray says. Sit-ups should be done with knees bent and arms crossed over the chest. Touch your elbows to your thighs. For people between ages 30 and 50, thirty sit-ups per minute is considered good for women, and thirty-five sit-ups per minute for men. For those 65 and older, fifteen is good for women and twenty-two for men. For 20-year-olds, thirty is good for women, and forty for men.

Push-ups are done with only hands and toes touching the floor. For people between 30 and 50, twenty push-ups per minute is good for women and twenty-three for men. For people 65 and older, thirteen is good for women and sixteen for men. For people in their twenties, twenty-two is good for women and thirty for men.

■ BODY COMPOSITION. To determine how much of your body is muscle and how much is fat, look in a mirror. "If you look fat," says McMurray, "you are fat." People who are overly fat should seek professional advice before starting an exercise program, he says.

After several months of regular exercise, says Abby King, most people find that simple tasks like running for a bus or doing work around the house become easier too. And that's when you know you're getting fit.

If you find yourself lacking in these areas, you should consult a physician or a physiotherapist.

A QUICK TEST FOR MACULAR DISEASE, THIEF OF CENTRAL VISION

One of the many eye disorders that can be conquered only with expanded research is macular degeneration (MD). The term MD actually encompasses a broad spectrum of diseases, all of which result in the same symptoms—loss of the central vision we use for reading, watching TV, driving, etc. Although MD affects primarily people over the age of 50, it is known to strike even children. It is estimated that 6 million people in the United States are victims.

Today, for certain types of MD, some treatment (called laser photocoagulation) is available to slow down, and in some cases even stop, the loss of vision if applied early in the course of the disease. Unfortunately for most MD victims no treatment is available. Only through additional research will appropriate treatments be found for this *and* the many other eye diseases afflicting humankind.

To see if you have early signs of MD, you can use the grid below as a quick screening test. Hold the page at a comfortable reading distance in good lighting. Wear your glasses if you normally do for

Figure 1

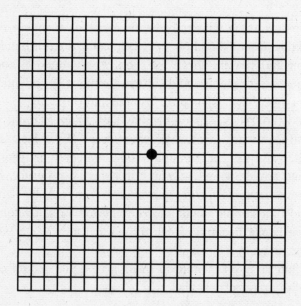

reading. First test one eye and then the other. Look at the dot in the center. If the straight lines appear blurred, bent, or twisted, you may be developing MD. If the lines appear distorted, consult your eye doctor as soon as possible to have a definitive examination.

GLAUCOMA: ARE YOU AT RISK?

Glaucoma is a group of diseases in which the pressure in the eye is higher than that particular eye can tolerate. The nerve fibers and blood vessels in the optic nerve become compressed and can be damaged or destroyed. For practical purposes, according to the New England Glaucoma Research Foundation in Boston, almost all glaucomas result from a decreased ability of fluid to leave the eye— the drainage mechanism is not working properly.

Although it is more common in adults than children, glaucoma can occur in people of all ages from birth to very advanced years; however, certain groups of people are known to be at somewhat higher risk of developing glaucoma than others. These are people who have a family history of glaucoma, people who are nearsighted or diabetic, people suffering from other diseases of the eye, and those who smoke.

Regular, professional eye exams are the best ways to detect the subtle, early-warning signs of glaucoma—the ultimate goal, of course, is to catch glaucoma in its earliest stages when it is easier to treat and before irreversible vision loss.

But here's a little test you can give yourself at home between eye exams, designed by George Spaeth, M.D., president of the American Glaucoma Society and director of glaucoma services at Wills Eye Hospital in Philadelphia.

1. Sit about a foot from a large TV.
2. Set it on a channel without a station—all you want is snow.
3. Close your left eye and look at the center of the screen with your right eye.

4. Are any areas of the screen blanked out, washed out, or less visible? Pay particular attention to the upper left-hand side of the screen. Diminished eyesight there may be caused by glaucoma.
5. Repeat with the other eye.

Now that you've taken the quiz, if you think you may have a problem, see a practitioner who can further and more comprehensively test your eyes and your vision.

HOW'S YOUR HEARING?

The Five-Minute Hearing Test below was field tested on seventy-one older patients in five cities; audiograms (tests where sounds are used to gauge your hearing ability) were also run on them. Results showed that the quiz worked; the people whose quiz scores indicated a need to see a physician were found to have a hearing impairment.

Mark the column that best describes the frequency with which you experience each situation or feeling.

■ SCORING

To calculate your score, give yourself 3 points for every time you checked the "Almost always" column, 2 for every "Half the time," 1 for every "Occasionally," and 0 for every "Never." If you have a blood relative who has a hearing loss, add another 3 points. Then total your points.

The American Academy of Otolaryngology—Head and Neck Surgery recommends the following:

0—5: Your hearing is fine. No action is required.

6—9: Suggest you see an ear-nose-and-throat (ENT) specialist.

10 and above: Strongly recommend you see a physician who specializes in hearing problems.

FIVE-MINUTE HEARING TEST

	ALMOST ALWAYS	HALF THE TIME	OCCASIONALLY	NEVER
1. I have a problem hearing over the telephone.				
2. I have trouble following the conversation when two or more people are talking at the same time.				
3. People complain that I turn the TV volume too high.				
4. I have to strain to understand conversations.				
5. I miss hearing some common sounds like the phone or doorbell ringing.				
6. I have trouble hearing conversations in a noisy background such as a party.				
7. I get confused about where sounds come from.				
8. I misunderstand some words in a sentence and need to ask people to repeat themselves.				
9. I especially have trouble understanding the speech of women and children.				
10. I have worked in noisy environments (assembly lines, jackhammers, jet engines, etc.).				
11. Many people I talk to seem to mumble (or don't speak clearly).				
12. People get annoyed because I misunderstand what they say.				
13. I misunderstand what others are saying and make inappropriate responses.				
14. I avoid social activities because I cannot hear well and fear I'll reply improperly.				
To be answered by a family member or friend: **15.** Do you think this person has a hearing loss?				

DO YOUR HEIGHT AND WEIGHT SEE EYE TO EYE?

The Metropolitan Life Insurance Company has been producing height and weight tables for many years. Reproduced below, the version in use today was updated and introduced in 1983. Before you check the table for your height and weight to see how closely you meet the guidelines, the first order of business is for you to determine whether you have a small, medium, or large frame.

What if the height and weight table indicates that you are 20 pounds overweight for your height? No doubt it's tempting to stand your ground *and* pronounce that, no, you're just a few inches shorter than you should be and that's not *your* fault. The fact of the matter is that this so-called discrepancy, based on Metropolitan Life's calculations, *does mean something*. You see, the 1983 Metropolitan Life height and weight table indicates the weights at which mortality is lowest—or longevity highest—and is intended to promote sound concepts of weight control. Simply put, the table indicates the weights at which people should live the longest. As the *Metropolitan Life Foundation Statistical Bulletin* (January–June 1983) phrases it: "[The table is] not used for underwriting or in the computation of premiums . . . [and is] not the weights that minimize illness or the incidence of disease. Neither [does it indicate] weights that optimize job performance, nor the weights for best appearance."

Indeed, Metropolitan Life avoids the words "ideal" or "desirable" when referring to the weight and height table, because these terms mean different things to different people, and different interpretations result only in confusion. The table's purpose, says the insurance company, is to serve as a health education tool, a guideline.

How then are these standards of weights calculated? Just like the earlier weight tables, the current one in use is based on extensive mortality studies of insured lives conducted by the Society of Actuaries and the Association of Life Insurance Medical Directors of America. In these studies people with major diseases such as heart disease, cancer, or diabetes were screened out to isolate the effect of weight on longevity. The 1983 figures indicate that today's adults can weigh more than their counterparts of two decades ago and "still anticipate favorable longevity," as the *Statistical Bulletin* puts it.

One more thing—though increased, the 1983 weights still fall below actual average weights. But Metropolitan Life concludes that the findings of earlier studies still apply—namely, that it is better to be lean than to be plump, and wiser to weigh less than the average rather than more.

MAKING AN APPROXIMATION OF YOUR FRAME SIZE

Extend your arm and bend the forearm upward at a 90-degree angle. Keep fingers straight and turn the inside of your wrist toward your body. If you have a caliper (a measuring instrument with two legs or jaws that can be adjusted to determine thickness), use it to measure the space between the two prominent bones on *either side* of your elbow. Without a caliper, place thumb and index finger of your other hand on these two bones. Measure the space between your fingers against a ruler or tape measure. Compare it with the data in the Approximation of Frame Size table, which lists elbow measurements for *medium-framed* men and women. Measurements lower than those listed indicate you have a small frame. Higher measurements indicate a large frame.

APPROXIMATION OF FRAME SIZE

HEIGHT IN 1″ HEELS	ELBOW BREADTH
Men	
5′2″–5′3″	2½″–2⅞″
5′4″–5′7″	2⅝″–2⅞″
5′8″–5′11″	2¾″–3″
6′0″–6′3″	2¾″–3⅛″
6′4″	2⅞″–3¼″
Women	
4′10″–4′11″	2¼″–2½″
5′0″–5′3″	2¼″–2½″
5′4″–5′7″	2⅜″–2⅝″
5′8″–5′11″	2⅜″–2⅝″
6′0″	2½″–2¾″

1983 METROPOLITAN
HEIGHT AND WEIGHT TABLE

MEN

| HEIGHT | | FRAME SIZE | | |
Feet	Inches	Small	Medium	Large
5	2	128–134	131–141	138–150
5	3	130–136	133–143	140–153
5	4	132–138	135–145	142–156
5	5	134–140	137–148	144–160
5	6	136–142	139–151	146–164
5	7	138–145	142–154	149–168
5	8	140–148	145–157	152–172
5	9	142–151	148–160	155–176
5	10	144–154	151–163	158–180
5	11	146–157	154–166	161–184
6	0	149–160	157–170	164–188
6	1	152–164	160–174	168–192
6	2	155–168	164–178	172–197
6	3	158–172	167–182	176–202
6	4	162–176	171–187	181–207

WOMEN

| HEIGHT | | FRAME SIZE | | |
Feet	Inches	Small	Medium	Large
4	10	102–111	109–121	118–131
4	11	103–113	111–123	120–134
5	0	104–115	113–126	122–137
5	1	106–118	115–129	125–140
5	2	108–121	118–132	128–143
5	3	111–124	121–135	131–147
5	4	114–127	124–138	134–151
5	5	117–130	127–141	137–155
5	6	120–133	130–144	140–159
5	7	123–136	133–147	143–163
5	8	126–139	136–150	146–167
5	9	129–142	139–153	149–170
5	10	132–145	142–156	152–173
5	11	135–148	145–159	155–176
6	0	138–151	148–162	158–179

Source of basic data: *Build Study*, 1979, Society of Actuaries and Association of Life Insurance Medical Directors of America, 1980.

Weights at ages 25–59 based on lowest mortality. Weight in pounds according to frame (in indoor clothing weighing 5 pounds for men and 3 pounds for women; shoes with 1-inch heels).

HOW TO DETERMINE YOUR TARGET HEART RATE

To get the maximum benefits from aerobic activity, it's necessary that you maintain a sufficiently high heart rate during your exercise to get a "training effect," or certain beneficial cardiovascular changes in the body. This is the concept of the "target heart rate"—the minimum rate at which your heart should be beating to get the optimum aerobic conditioning effect.

Dr. Kenneth Cooper's aerobic point system, reproduced below, is structured in such a way that, if you earn a minimum number of points per week, you'll get an adequate training effect without having to worry about what your heart rate is during exercise. But there are a number of new aerobic activities, like aerobic dancing and roller skating, which are sometimes hard to quantify in terms of aerobic points.

So, because you may be interested in working these activities into your personal exercise program, it's important for you to understand how the target heart rate concept works. Then, even if you haven't been able to set up an aerobic point chart for the form of exercise you have chosen, you'll still be able to evaluate whether or not this activity will help achieve aerobic conditioning.

Here's an easy procedure to determine your personal target heart rate. First, determine your resting heart rate. To get this figure, monitor your pulse at the wrist, at the neck, or by placing your hand over your heart. Count every beat for 15 seconds, and then multiply that figure by 4 to get the number of heartbeats per minute.

If you measure the number of beats for a shorter period than 15 seconds—say 6 or 10 seconds—the possibility of committing a major error is greatly magnified. For example, if you're off one beat over a 15-second period, you'll only be off four beats over the 1-minute period. But if you make one error during a 6-second count, your error over the minute period could be plus or minus ten heartbeats.

Finally, Cooper recommends that you take your heart rate at the heart itself or the wrist, rather than at the carotid artery at the neck. The reason for this is that some studies have shown that, if you press too hard on the neck, you may actually slow down your rate by as much as three to four beats per minute.

For the purpose of illustrating the way to calculate your target heart rate, let's assume for the rest of this discussion that you are a 50-year-old man or woman.

Next, use the appropriate formula. For men: Predicted Maximum Heart Rate (PMHR) = 205 minus half your age. For women: PMHR = 220 minus age. For example, at 50 years of age, a man's predicted maximum heart rate would be 205 minus 25 = 180. For women, it would be 220 minus 50 = 170.

The third step is a rather simple calculation: Take 80 percent of 180, and get 144 beats per minute. If your heart rate exceeds that figure for a minimum of 20 minutes, four times per week, then you will get an aerobic training effect. In fact, combinations of a heart rate of 130 for 30 minutes, or 150 for 10 minutes, four times a week, will in general give you the same results.

Finally, there is the problem of how to *monitor* your heart rate accurately during exercise to be sure you're reaching your target heart rate and getting the full aerobic benefits. The problem here is that it usually takes at least 20 seconds to take your pulse after you stop exercising. That includes 5 to 10 seconds just to find the pulse, waiting a few seconds for the second hand to be just right, and then another 10 seconds to count the beats.

In addition, if you are in good condition, your heart rate may drop at a rate of a beat per minute for the first 15 to 20 seconds after exercise. So it's necessary to correct your reading upward to find your true heart rate during exercise. The technique Cooper suggests for the highly conditioned person is to go ahead and take your pulse rate within 20 seconds after you stop your aerobic exercise. Then, add 10 percent to this pulse rate to get your heart rate during exercise. For example, if you counted a heart rate of 160, in reality it was probably 10 percent higher at maximum, or 176.

PREDICTED MAXIMUM HEART RATES
ADJUSTED FOR AGE AND FITNESS

AGE	VERY POOR AND POOR	FAIR	GOOD AND EXCELLENT	AGE	VERY POOR AND POOR	FAIR	GOOD AND EXCELLENT
20	201	201	196	45	174	183	183
21	199	200	196	46	173	182	183
22	198	199	195	47	172	181	182
23	197	198	195	48	171	181	182
24	196	198	194	49	170	180	181
25	195	197	194	50	168	179	180
26	194	196	193	51	167	179	180
27	193	196	193	52	166	178	179
28	192	195	192	53	165	177	179
29	191	193	192	54	164	176	178
30	190	193	191	55	163	176	178
31	189	193	191	56	162	175	177
32	188	192	190	57	161	174	177
33	187	191	189	58	160	174	176
34	186	191	189	59	159	173	176
35	184	190	188	60	158	172	175
36	183	189	188	61	157	172	175
37	182	189	187	62	156	171	174
38	181	188	187	63	155	170	174
39	180	187	186	64	154	169	173
40	179	186	186	65	152	169	173
41	178	186	185	66	151	168	172
42	177	185	185	67	150	167	171
43	176	184	184	68	149	167	171
44	175	184	184	69	148	166	170
				70	147	165	170

Note: If the level of fitness is unknown prior to stress testing, use the "Fair" category.

HOW TO DO BREAST SELF-EXAMINATION

Here is one of the best ways to protect yourself from breast cancer and put your mind at ease. The other two ways are a breast exam by a doctor or someone trained to do it and a breast X ray (mammogram).

Why do the breast self-exam? There are many good reasons for doing the breast self-exam (BSE) each month. One reason is that breast cancer is most easily treated and cured when it is found early. Another is that, if you do BSE every month, it will increase your skill and confidence. When you get to know how your breasts normally feel, you will quickly be able to feel any change. Another reason—it's easy to do. Remember: BSE could save your breast—and save your life. Most breast lumps are found by women themselves, but, in fact, most lumps in the breast are not cancer. Be safe, be sure.

When to do BSE? The best time to do BSE is about a week after your period, when breasts are not tender or swollen. If you do not have regular periods or sometimes skip a month, do BSE on the same day every month.

Now, how to do BSE.

1. Lie down and put a pillow under your left shoulder. Place your left arm behind your head. (Figure 2a, page 89.)
2. Use the finger pads of your three middle fingers on your right hand to feel for lumps. Your finger pads are the top third of each finger. (Figure 2b.)
3. Press firmly enough to know how your breast feels. If you're not sure how hard to press, ask your doctor or nurse. Or try to copy the way your doctor uses the finger pads during a breast exam. Learn what your breast feels like most of the time. A firm ridge in the lower curve of each breast is normal.
4. Move around the breast in a set way. You can choose either the circle, the up-and-down line, or the wedge. Do it the same way every time. It will help you to make sure that you've gone over the entire breast area, and to remember how your breast feels each month.
5. Now examine your right breast, using left-hand finger pads.
6. If you find any changes, see your doctor right away.

■ FOR ADDED SAFETY

You might want to check your breasts while standing in front of a mirror, right after you do your BSE each month. See if there are any changes in the way your breasts look, dimpling of the skin, or changes in the nipple, redness, or swelling. You might also want to do an extra BSE while you're in the shower. Your soapy hands will glide over the wet skin, making it easy to check how your breasts feel. (Figure 2c.)

Figure 2

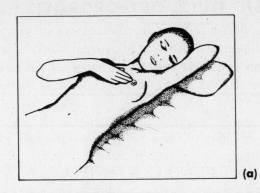

(a)

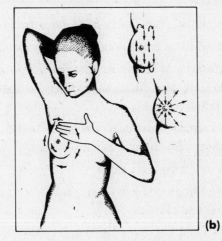

(b)

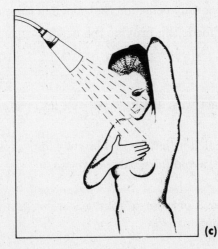

(c)

HEALTH IQ QUIZ: OSTEOPOROSIS

Nearly 20 million Americans are affected by osteoporosis each year. Medical professionals have determined that exercise, along with adequate calcium, can help reduce your chances of getting osteoporosis.

Check your Health IQ on osteoporosis by taking the quiz below. True or false:

1. Women are more likely than men to break bones as they grow older.

2. There are things you can do to prevent or slow down osteoporosis.

3. Women lose bone mass faster after menopause.

4. White women have more bone mass than black women.

5. A drop in estrogen levels in the years just after menopause contributes to women being more likely to break bones in their wrist or spine than men.

6. There is no simple, low-cost screening test for accurately detecting osteoporosis before a bone breaks.

7. X rays can measure bone mass.

8. Many of the things you can do to prevent osteoporosis are also used to treat the disease.

9. Most adults need between 1,000 and 1,500 mg of calcium each day and generally consume that much in their diet.

10. Only dairy foods can provide the needed calcium.

■ ANSWERS

1. True.
   Women start with about 30 percent less bone mass than men.
2. True.
   Increase calcium intake, avoid smoking, avoid heavy alcohol use, exercise, avoid falls, take estrogen.
3. True.
   About 2 to 3 percent a year, occurring the first five to ten years after menopause.

4. False.

5. True.

This usually occurs from ages 45 to 60.

6. True.

However, a physician may use a number of tests to check your risk, starting with a medical history. A physical exam and blood and urine tests may help rule out other diseases that weaken bone.

7. True.

But simple X rays do not show bone loss until it is advanced. Some other methods are unable to measure bone mass in certain parts of the body. Some methods that are used, however, are photo absorptiometry (a scanning method for measuring bone density) and computed axial tomography, or CAT scan (a highly sophisticated, cross-sectional X ray).

8. True.

9. False.

Most adults get only about 500 mg of calcium a day.

10. False.

Calcium supplements can help make up for the calcium you don't get in food. Some people do not like or cannot eat dairy foods.

A SELF-EXAM FOR TESTICULAR CANCER

Men have finally discovered something women have known for quite some time—the value of self-examination for cancer. Women have learned to do self-examination for breast cancer, and it has paid off in the number of cancers that have been detected early. Cancer experts tell us that early detection of cancer leads to early treatment and increased chances of survival.

This is especially true when dealing with testicular cancer, a form of male cancer that can be detected through self-examination. However, it's not something that gets the media attention given to breast cancer, lung cancer, or colon cancer, nor is it usually the topic of male conversation. A lot of this has to do with ignorance of both the existence of testicular cancer *and* the potentially lifesaving procedure. But there also may be embarrassment, fear, and perhaps even unwillingness on the part of men to admit that something could threaten their sexuality and fertility. Nonetheless, testicular cancer is a fact of life.

At one time a confirmed diagnosis meant almost certain death, but today—with early detection—the recovery rate is roughly 90 percent. Testicular cancer victims are most often between the ages of 15 and 35, with approximately 5,000 new cases reported every year. For some unknown reason, white men are four times more likely to develop the disease than black men. According to one study, it is responsible for one in seven cancer deaths in this age group.

Most tumors found in the testicles are malignant and spread rapidly; in half of all cases, the cancer invades other parts of the body, usually the lungs or abdominal lymph tissue. Because doctors are concerned with the spread of cancer cells throughout the body, they aggressively pursue the cancer with surgery, radiation, and chemotherapy. You may avoid subjecting yourself to such an ordeal by learning a simple self-exam technique.

Examining yourself for testicular cancer is relatively easy and doesn't require more than three minutes of your time once a month. Every man should be able to spare that for this important health check. Here's how to get started:

1. It's best to do the exam following a warm bath or shower.
2. Make sure the scrotal skin is relaxed.
3. Examine one testicle at a time.
4. Roll each testicle between the thumb and fingers of both hands.
5. Massage the surface lightly and check for any irregularities or anything that seems strange (you may feel the epididymis, which runs up the back of the testicle, but that's normal).
6. If you find any bumps or hard lumps, contact your doctor.

VASECTOMY MYTHS:
HOW MANY HAVE YOU FALLEN FOR?

The decision to have a vasectomy is often made more difficult by the nagging suspicion that maybe—just maybe—there's more than fertility at stake here.

Men who are willing to surrender their ability to father children can't help but wonder if the deal might somehow entail other, unwanted aftereffects. Vague fears of unknown, irreversible threats to their future health and sexuality often cloud their perception of the procedure.

And of course, you can always find someone who's more than willing to make up outrageous outcomes and insist that these dire consequences of vasectomy are absolute, irrefutable scientific truth.

(These tend to be the same people who know for a fact that Elvis once fathered a two-headed baby who is currently being trained to sing duets, and that our government is hiding the bodies of hundreds of crash-landed aliens in a secret warehouse in Sacramento.)

But even the realization that these worst-case medical opinions are coming from someone who also claims to know Bigfoot personally may not be all that reassuring when you're in the vulnerable position of trying to decide if such a sensitive procedure is really for you.

Want to know just how up you are on the real facts? Test yourself with this quiz, originally put together (in a slightly different form) for physicians by Sumner Marshall, M.D., a clinical professor of urology at the University of California Medical Center, San Francisco.

Dr. Marshall, and the editors of the journal *Medical Aspects of Human Sexuality*, where Dr. Marshall's original, physician-oriented quiz first appeared, have been kind enough to allow us to adapt the questions and answers into less-medical language. True or false:

1. A vasectomy is often followed by decreased sex drive and an impaired ability to get erections.

2. Following a vasectomy, there is an increased chance of developing cardiovascular (heart) disease.

3. Having a vasectomy disrupts your immune system, causing an increased risk of autoimmune diseases like multiple sclerosis, rheumatoid arthritis, and certain forms of cancer.

4. Vasectomized men experience a marked decrease in the amount of fluid they ejaculate.

5. It is safe to stop using other forms of contraception (birth control) six weeks after a vasectomy.

6. If a woman gets pregnant a year after her partner's vasectomy, and tests of her partner's semen show no sperm, she must have had intercourse with another man.

7. Men should consider vasectomies irreversible.

■ ANSWERS

1. False.

Actually, most men report an increase in sex drive, which may be due to the psychological relief of not having to worry about supporting any future children. And a vasectomy has no effect on hormonal function, so it doesn't hinder your ability to have erections.

2. False.

Studies have found increased cholesterol levels in vasectomized monkeys, but this increase has not been found in studies of vasectomized men. Some individuals may experience an increase in cholesterol levels after a vasectomy, but the same would probably be true after any type of operation. Studies of students taking exams suggest that emotional stress itself—such as that caused by undergoing surgery—may cause a temporary elevation of blood cholesterol levels.

3. False.

This misconception is based on the elevated levels of sperm antibodies that are often found after vasectomy. While these increased antibody levels do develop in a high percentage of vasectomized men, no evidence exists that they cause any kind of disease.

4. False.

More than 99 percent of the fluid that men ejaculate comes from the prostate and seminal vesicles—areas that are still connected after the vasectomy. Less than 1 percent of the ejaculate comes from the area that has been closed off—the testicles themselves. Since that sperm-containing 1 percent is almost too small an amount to be noticed, a vasectomy causes no real decrease in the volume of fluid that's ejaculated.

5. False.

No more sperm can come up from the testicles themselves after a vasectomy, but a sperm reservoir located beyond the testicles (and past the site of the vasectomy) must still be emptied before the ejaculate will be totally free of active sperm.

The length of time this takes varies from man to man. One review of 200 consecutive cases found that as many as ten ejaculations are frequently necessary before the fluid becomes completely sperm-free. However, a man should not be considered medically sterile until he has had a minimum of sixteen ejaculations after a vasectomy, with the last two of those being certified sperm-free by strict testing.

There is also the possibility (although it's rare) of the part that's severed during the vasectomy (the vas deferens) spontaneously reconnecting. Since this is most likely to occur within the first two months after vasectomy (again, if it happens at all), it's advisable to wait three to four months before having unprotected intercourse.

6. False.

There is always the possibility that a man's sperm may re-emerge after vasectomy. The vas deferens may spontaneously reconnect, or the man may have been told his sperm reservoir was empty before it actually was, due to a mistaken interpretation of a test (reading an active sperm sample as negative).

Even a sperm test taken after the pregnancy has been discovered that shows no active sperm is not proof of another man's involvement. Active sperm could well have been present when the woman became pregnant months before. Men who deny the possibility of their fertility in such a situation are not only medically incorrect; they also risk destroying the relationship in question.

7. Partially true.

Essentially, a man should not have a vasectomy if he has any thoughts that he might want to reverse the procedure in the future. Current surgical techniques do make successful reversal possible, particularly if the decision to reverse is made within five years of the vasectomy, and the previous surgery has not caused scar tissue to develop. Nevertheless, most physicians strongly advise against a vasectomy in situations where a man may someday want to father more children, or where childbearing plans might change.

THE ROCKPORT FITNESS WALKING TEST

Walking is arguably the best form of exercise you can undertake. Aerobically speaking, it may be the world's most underrated sport. And you can burn more calories by brisk walking than by jogging.

CALORIES

Fitness Walking	**248**
Tennis (vigorous singles)	**311**
Moderate Fitness Walking up a mild incline (5%)	**338**
Light Jogging (5.5 mph)	**455**
Brisk Fitness Walking up a moderate incline (10%)	**541**

It's pretty tough to hurt yourself walking. Runners land with three or four times their body weight every time their feet hit the ground. Walkers, by way of contrast, land with only one to one-and-a-half times their body weight. Walking exercises muscles all over your body, and it is actually one of the best exercises for healthy feet.

Walking is great exercise for people who are in terrific shape.

And it's just as good for people in lousy shape. Virtually every cardiac rehabilitation program in America bases its exercise regimen on *walking*.

Seventy-seven million Americans walk as their exercise of choice. If you haven't already joined the fun, chances are you will.

The Rockport Fitness Walking Test is a series of fitness walking programs—tests designed to improve your cardiovascular health. Whether you walk outside, on a track, or on a treadmill, the Rockport Fitness Walking Test can change your entire perspective on physical fitness. Over the next twenty weeks, you can lose weight and tone muscles all over your body. The five programs listed in this quiz are more than sufficient to provide the focus you need to follow a thorough and extremely rewarding exercise regimen that you can continue for the rest of your life.

Before we proceed, a brief word of caution: While the Rockport Fitness Walking Test has no significant limitations in terms of vigor, ease, familiarity, or injury risk, *no* exercise test or program should be undertaken without the consent of your personal physician.

The Rockport Fitness Walking Test is based on your pulse—a fundamental rhythm of your body. The following programs can be distilled into one key question: *How fast does your heart beat at a given level of exertion?*

PRETEST WARM-UP

1. Take your pulse. Before you actually take the test, you need to know how to take your pulse accurately. If you do not already know how to do this, here is an easy way to learn. Walk in place for 30 seconds and then gently put your second and third fingers together (don't use your thumb) on your radial artery just inside the wrist bone. You can also take your pulse on the side of your neck at the level of the Adam's apple, just below the jaw, on your temple, or over your heart. Count your pulse for 15 seconds (but no more) and multiply by four to determine your pulse per minute.

2. Find a measured track or measure out a mile on your own. Most

high schools and recreation facilities have a quarter-mile track. If you measure out on your own—by using your car's odometer, for instance—do it on a flat road with as few interruptions (e.g., stoplights) as possible.

THE ROCKPORT FITNESS WALKING TEST

1. Walk one mile as fast as you can. Stretch for 5 to 10 minutes before and after. Wear good walking shoes and loose-fitting clothes, and maintain a steady pace.
2. Record your time. Do this to the nearest second. Most people walk between 3.0 and 6.0 miles per hour, so it should take 10 to 20 minutes to walk the mile.
3. Record your heart rate immediately at the end of the mile (it begins to slow almost immediately after you stop walking). Count your pulse for 15 seconds and multiply by four, then record this number. This gives you your heart rate per minute after your test walk.

FINDING YOUR FITNESS LEVEL

1. Look at the Rockport Fitness Walking Test charts, according to the fitness norms established by the American Heart Association. Locate the appropriate Relative Fitness Level chart for your age and sex.
2. Mark the point on the chart defined by your walking time and heart rate at the end of the walk. This point allows you to compare your performance to that of others in your age and sex category.
3. Next, look at the appropriate Exercise Program chart for your age and sex. Again, mark your coordinates on this chart. Note the level you fall in.
4. Begin your twenty-week fitness walking program. Turn to the program sheet that corresponds to the level you were in on the Exercise Program chart. Start the program outlined for your level and follow it for twenty weeks.

5. Repeat the Rockport Fitness Walking Test at the end of the twenty weeks. This determines your fitness level and recommends a new fitness walking program.

RELATIVE FITNESS LEVEL CHARTS

These charts are designed to tell you how fit you are compared to other individuals of your age and sex. For example, if your coordinates place you in the "above average" section of the chart, you're in better shape than the average person in your category.

The charts are based on weights of 170 pounds for men and 125 pounds for women. If you weigh substantially less, your relative cardiovascular fitness level will be slightly underestimated. Conversely, if you weigh substantially more, your cardiovascular fitness will be slightly overestimated.

THE

ROCKPORT FITNESS

WALKING TEST

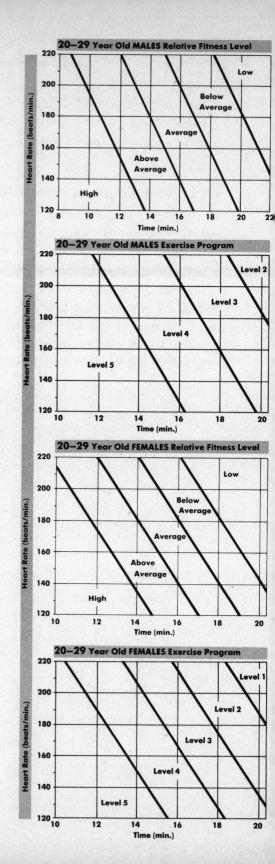

20–29 Year Old MALES Relative Fitness Level

Heart Rate (beats/min.)

Low

Below Average

Average

Above Average

High

Time (min.)

20–29 Year Old MALES Exercise Program

Heart Rate (beats/min.)

Level 2

Level 3

Level 4

Level 5

Time (min.)

20–29 Year Old FEMALES Relative Fitness Level

Heart Rate (beats/min.)

Low

Below Average

Average

Above Average

High

Time (min.)

20–29 Year Old FEMALES Exercise Program

Heart Rate (beats/min.)

Level 1

Level 2

Level 3

Level 4

Level 5

Time (min.)

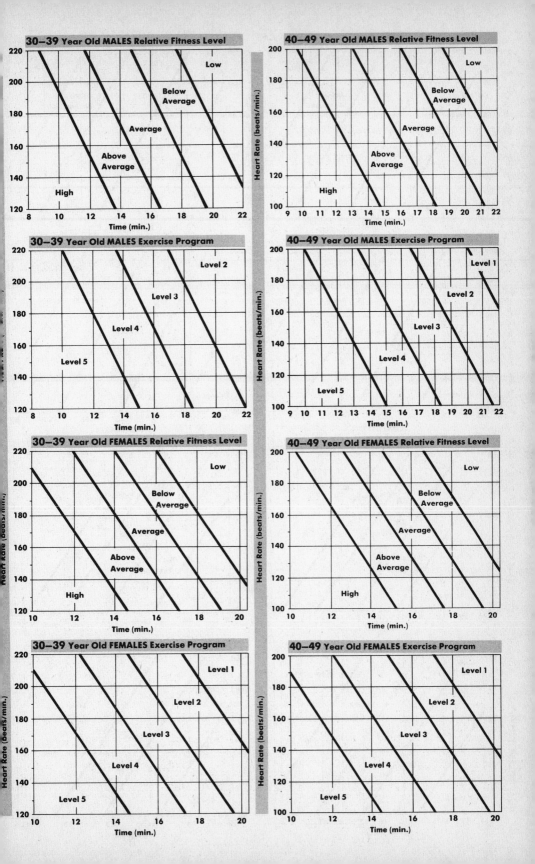

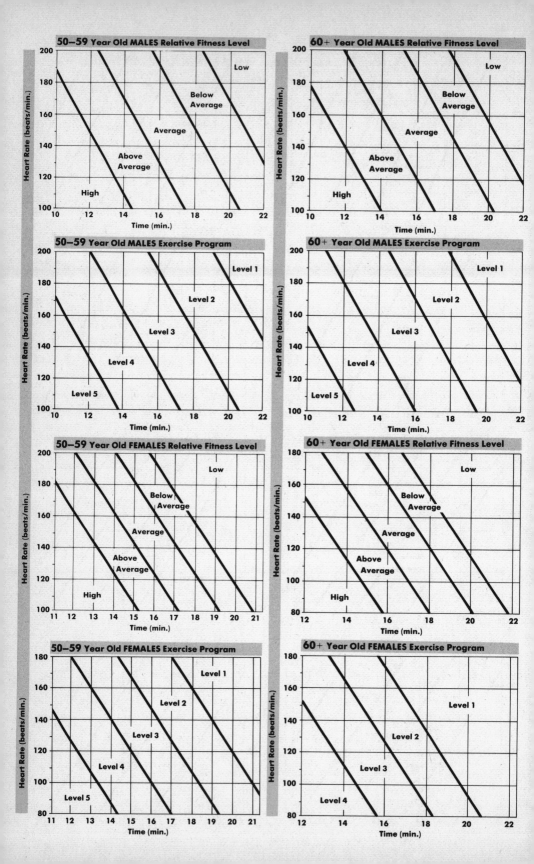

EXERCISE PROGRAMS

The programs outlined on the following pages were developed by the cardiologists and exercise physiologists from the Exercise Physiology and Nutrition Lab and Department of Exercise Science at the University of Massachusetts Medical School, using extensive field data. They are designed to help maintain or improve your level of fitness, depending on your current level. For optimal results, follow the programs closely.

At the end of the twenty-week period, retake the Rockport Fitness Walking Test to determine your new fitness level and exercise program.

On each program there are lines labeled Pace and Heart Rate. The pace listed is only an approximation. Walking speed should be determined by the pace that keeps your heart rate at the appropriate percentage of maximum listed. To determine your maximum heart rate, subtract your age from 220.

EXERCISE PROGRAMS

LEVEL 1

WEEK	1–2	3–4	5	6	7–8	9	10	11	12–13	14	15–16	17–18	19–20*
WARM-UP (mins. before walk stretches)	5–7	5–7	5–7	5–7	5–7	5–7	5–7	5–7	5–7	5–7	5–7	5–7	5–7
MILEAGE	1.0	1.25	1.5	1.5	1.75	2.0	2.0	2.0	2.25	2.5	2.5	2.75	3.0
PACE (mph)	3.0	3.0	3.0	3.5	3.5	3.5	3.75	3.75	3.75	3.75	4.0	4.0	4.0
HEART RATE (% of max)	60	60	60	60–70	60–70	60–70	60–70	70	70	70	70	70–80	70–80
COOLDOWN (mins. after walk stretches)	5–7	5–7	5–7	5–7	5–7	5–7	5–7	5–7	5–7	5–7	5–7	5–7	5–7
FREQUENCY (times per week)	5	5	5	5	5	5	5	5	5	5	5	5	5

LEVEL 2

WEEK	1–2	3–4	5–6	7	8–9	10–12	13	14	15–16	17–18	19–20†
WARM-UP (mins. before walk stretches)	5–7	5–7	5–7	5–7	5–7	5–7	5–7	5–7	5–7	5–7	5–7
MILEAGE	1.5	1.75	2.0	2.0	2.25	2.5	2.75	2.75	3.0	3.25	3.5
PACE (mph)	3.0	3.0	3.0	3.5	3.5	3.5	3.5	4.0	4.0	4.0	4.0
HEART RATE (% of max)	60–70	60–70	60–70	70	70	70	70	70–80	70–80	70–80	70–80
COOLDOWN (mins. after walk stretches)	5–7	5–7	5–7	5–7	5–7	5–7	5–7	5–7	5–7	5–7	5–7
FREQUENCY (times per week)	5	5	5	5	5	5	5	5	5	5	5

LEVEL 3

WEEK	1	2	3-4	5	6-8	9-10	11-12	13-14	15	16-17	18-20‡
WARM-UP (mins. before walk stretches)	5-7	5-7	5-7	5-7	5-7	5-7	5-7	5-7	5-7	5-7	5-7
MILEAGE	2.0	2.25	2.5	2.75	2.75	3.0	3.0	3.25	3.5	3.5	4.0
PACE (mph)	3.0	3.0	3.0	3.0	3.5	3.5	4.0	4.0	4.0	4.5	4.5
HEART RATE (% of max)	70	70	70	70	70	70	70-80	70-80	70-80	70-80	70-80
COOLDOWN (mins. after walk stretches)	5-7	5-7	5-7	5-7	5-7	5-7	5-7	5-7	5-7	5-7	5-7
FREQUENCY (times per week)	5	5	5	5	5	5	5	5	5	5	5

LEVEL 4

WEEK	1	2	3-4	5	6	7	8	9-10	11-14	15-20§
WARM-UP (mins. before walk stretches)	5-7	5-7	5-7	5-7	5-7	5-7	5-7	5-7	5-7	5-7
MILEAGE	2.5	2.75	3.0	3.25	3.25	3.5	3.75	4.0	4.0	4.0
PACE (mph)	3.5	3.5	3.5	3.5	4.0	4.0	4.0	4.0	4.5	4.5
INCLINE/WEIGHT										+
HEART RATE (% of max)	70	70	70	70	70-80	70-80	70-80	70-80	70-80	70-80
COOLDOWN (mins. after walk stretches)	5-7	5-7	5-7	5-7	5-7	5-7	5-7	5-7	5-7	5-7
FREQUENCY (times per week)	5	5	5	5	5	5	5	5	5	3

LEVEL 5

WEEK	1	2	3	4	5	6	7–20[||]
WARM-UP (mins. before walk stretches)	5–7	5–7	5–7	5–7	5–7	5–7	5–7
MILEAGE	3.0	3.25	3.5	3.5	3.75	4.0	4.0
PACE (mph)	4.0	4.0	4.0	4.5	4.5	4.5	4.5
INCLINE/WEIGHT							+
HEART RATE (% of max)	70	70	70	70–80	70–80	70–80	70–80
COOLDOWN (mins. after walk stretches)	5–7	5–7	5–7	5–7	5–7	5–7	5–7
FREQUENCY (times per week)	5	5	5	5	5	5	3

LEVEL 3 MAINTENANCE PROGRAM

WARM-UP: 5–7 minutes before walk stretches

AEROBIC WORKOUT: mileage: 4.0 pace: 4.5 mph

HEART RATE: 70–80% of maximum

COOLDOWN: 5–7 minutes after walk stretches

FREQUENCY: 3–5 times per week

WEEKLY MILEAGE: 12–20 miles

LEVELS 4 AND 5 MAINTENANCE PROGRAM

WARM-UP: 5–7 minutes before walk stretches

AEROBIC WORKOUT: mileage: 4.0 pace: 4.5 mph
weight/incline: add weights to upper body or add hill walking as needed to keep heart rate in target zone (70–80% of predicted maximum).

HEART RATE: 70–80% of maximum

COOLDOWN: 5–7 minutes after walk stretches

FREQUENCY: 3–5 times per week

WEEKLY MILEAGE: 12–20 miles

*At the end of the twenty-week fitness walking protocol, retest yourself to establish your new program.

†At the end of the twenty-week fitness walking protocol, retest yourself to establish your new program.

‡At the end of the twenty-week fitness walking protocol, you may either retest yourself and move to a new fitness walking category or follow the Level 3 Maintenance Program for a lifetime of fitness walking.

§At the end of the twenty-week fitness walking protocol, follow the Levels 4/5 Maintenance Program for a lifetime of fitness walking.

‖At the end of the twenty-week fitness walking protocol, turn to the Levels 4/5 Maintenance Program for a lifetime of fitness walking.

4. HOW'S YOUR CHILD?

Protecting the health of their child is usually the first priority of parents. In fact, the very process of parenting is designed to ensure the successful and safe passage from childhood to adulthood.

In this chapter, we provide a group of tests that are designed to help you better observe and intervene in your child's health and safety. We also provide a test that will give you greater insight into your rights when it comes to your child's health. This latter test has surprised many a parent.

Many of us assume that what is good for us adults is good for our kids. Often that is not the case. Take diet, for instance. Are the foods you eat the best ones for your child? Or what about fitness? Is your child getting the proper amount and right types of exercise? Have you ever taken a close look at the playground your child uses? Is it safe for someone in his or her age range?

Your child relies on you to oversee his or her health. The tests in this chapter are meant to give you greater skills and insight in fulfilling your responsibilities.

WHAT'S YOUR PARENTING QUOTIENT?

Being a good parent is more than liking tiny people and having an ample bank account. The best of intentions need to be grounded in some sophistication about this most important and least understood of all jobs.

Can a quiz like this one help you see just how fit you are for the vocation? Not really. But you may find it fun, and along the way you'll pick up a couple of facts—or well-documented opinions, at any rate.

You needn't limit yourself to one best answer. Once you've finished, check yourself against our answers. Scoring is figured at the end of the test.

1. All parents want their children to be well-liked. Your best strategy is to
   (a) encourage your kids to have as many friends as possible, because a broad social universe helps ensure they'll be well-adjusted adults.
   (b) let them decide how many or how few friends to have.
   (c) suggest they have only a few, carefully selected friends in order to discourage superficial behavior in dealing with other people.
   (d) set a goal for your children, for instance, of one-and-a-half close friends for each year of age.

2. When kids spend time watching a weekly series on network television, chances are good that their minds
   (a) will vegetate, because television viewing by definition is a passive way in which to spend time.
   (b) may be stretched by learning to follow the ambiguities and subplots now found in the more creative shows.

(c) will shrink up to 5 percent by volume.

(d) are given a good workout because the eyes must contend with sixteen frames of visual information each second.

3. Children seem to absorb everything they see on the television screen. In fact, disturbing shows

(a) have been found to go in one ear and out the other, because even the youngest of children realize that what comes out of a little box can't be real.

(b) are no more troubling to a child than storybooks.

(c) are considered to be reality by very young children.

(d) are not taken as reality by older children, but are regarded as representing the way things probably are in real life.

4. Stress is quite familiar among adults. Children experience stress, too,

(a) and can learn problem-solving techniques that will enable them to work out troubles on their own.

(b) but only after entering their teens; younger kids have been found to enjoy a built-in protection from true psychological stress.

(c) but at such a deep, unconscious level that only a trained therapist should try to intervene.

(d) and their dreams and fantasies will do the important work of resolving these problems, naturally and without help from adults.

5. Which of the following is the best description of the cause of a young child's temper tantrum?

(a) an exceptionally intense, although temporary, hatred for one or both parents

(b) sensory overload, thanks to our culture's information explosion

(c) a powerful sense of independence

(d) a feeling of despair at not being able to arrange life in a way he or she wants

6. Which of the following is a sign that a child may be "gifted"?

(a) cooperation and dependability

(b) sense of humor

(c) candidness

(d) energy and good health

(e) high scores on intelligence tests

7. A young child's fantasies
    (a) are a warning sign to alert knowledgeable parents that a full-blown neurosis may soon follow.
    (b) are harmless enough, because they don't involve him or her on an emotional level.
    (c) should be encouraged and praised at every possible opportunity.
    (d) are a telltale sign the child isn't getting enough fantasy material through educational toys and quality television programming.
    (e) are an invaluable part of his or her development, and time should be allowed for them to happen on their own.

8. Almost every family owns at least one hand-held calculator. To encourage a child to learn mathematics skills, parents should
    (a) keep these easy-to-use crutches out of a child's hands.
    (b) rely on the schools to introduce the child to calculators as they see fit.
    (c) come up with daily ways for the child to use a calculator at home.
    (d) invest in a good-quality abacus and ask the child to use this time-tested instrument instead.

9. When a child in kindergarten or first grade complains repeatedly of a stomachache as an excuse to keep from going to school, he or she is probably
    (a) responding to a real pain caused by mental stress.
    (b) eating Cheez-Whiz out of the jar.
    (c) making it up.
    (d) troubled by a purely physical ailment.

10. When the Educational Testing Service looked into the back-

grounds of gifted high school girls, it found that important playtime factors included

(a) dolls.

(b) construction toys, Legos in particular.

(c) "tomboy" activities such as tree climbing and building forts.

(d) microscopes and chemistry sets.

11. According to a recent British study of girls between the ages of 12 and 18, most of those who see themselves as being overweight

    (a) would benefit from dieting.

    (b) are mistaken.

    (c) have simply made the fashion blunder of wearing clothes with horizontal stripes.

    (d) will tend to become more accepting of their weight as they go through their teens.

12. Adults need anywhere from 6 to 10 hours of sleep per day, on average. Kids between ages 2 and 5 need

    (a) 8 or 9 hours.

    (b) 11 or 12 hours.

    (c) more than 13 hours.

13. The traditional wisdom that kids should eat a good breakfast before school

    (a) has been discounted as an old-wives' tale, because the brain is now known to be relatively immune to short-term lapses in nutrition.

    (b) was recently revealed to be a fiction perpetrated by major cereal companies, according to a U.S. Senate subcommittee.

    (c) has a basis in recent findings that show the brain is surprisingly sensitive to fluctuations of nutrient intake.

    (d) has sadly resulted in a generation of chubby children.

14. Spats are as common among siblings as freckles and cowlicks. But some pairings are apt to be stormier than others. Which of the following sibling relationships produces the most violent verbal and emotional attacks?

(a) between a girl and her older sister.

(b) between a boy and his older brother.

(c) between a boy and his older sister.

(d) between a girl and her older brother.

15. The newborn's world can best be described as

    (a) a "booming, buzzing confusion," in the words of William James.

    (b) a comatose state, in which eyes and ears are nearly inoperable.

    (c) one in which colors, forms, patterns, and faces can be perceived.

    (d) a round-the-clock thirst.

16. There is a trend for school counselors to become more involved with helping individual children with their emotional problems. This new breed of counselors has found that young children

    (a) have fewer defenses, and therefore tend to express themselves more freely than adults.

    (b) sadly do not yet have the verbal skills necessary to describe their emotional world.

    (c) are too emotionally unformed to handle the traumas that inevitably surface in a one-on-one session.

    (d) simply are too physically active to remain prone on the counselor's couch for 40 minutes.

■ ANSWERS

1. (b) Zick Rubin cautions in *Children's Friendships* (Harvard University Press, 1980) that "adults should respect the real differences between children that motivate some to establish relations with many others, some to concentrate on one or two close friendships, and some to spend a good deal of time by themselves." So don't feel there is some sort of friendship quota that is best for your kids. "Any of these patterns may be satisfying and appropriate for a particular child," Dr. Rubin assures parents.

2. (b) Network TV may still be a "vast wasteland," as FCC chairman Newton Minow labeled it in the early 1960s. But there are oases of quality that parents should be alert for, according to Patricia Marks Greenfield in her book *Mind and Media* (Harvard University Press, 1984).

No matter what your children watch, you can add another level of interest and complexity by making comments and asking questions during worthwhile shows. In particular, by discussing televised material on sex roles, violence, and commercialism, you can help prepare your children for handling the influence of this powerful medium.

3. (c) and (d) Children deal differently with television as they grow older. The very young "equate all of television except cartoons with reality," according to Patricia Marks Greenfield. As they grow older, they're better able to discriminate between fact and fiction; nonetheless, she says, they continue to "believe that what they see on television represents something that *probably* happens in the real world."

Answer (b) is not correct, because television has been found to come closer than books in creating an illusion of reality.

4. (a) Even though no period of life is immune to stress, adults may be too quick to dismiss a child's withdrawal or acting up as just an inevitable stage of growing up.

Parents can help children as young as four to resolve their own stressful problems through a simple problem-solving technique, according to Avis Brenner, Ed.D., in *Helping Your Children Cope with Stress* (Lexington Books, 1984). She says a child first should be trained to come up with alternate solutions to a problem, and then to think through the consequences of each solution.

5. (d) It can be hard to keep from taking a child's temper tantrum personally, as suggested in (a). But Dr. Bruno Bettelheim, author of many books on the psychology of children, says that these outbursts are directed inward. In his guide to child-rearing, *A Good Enough Parent* (Alfred A. Knopf, 1987), he

explains that a young child believes he or she does not have "a self that works for him" and experiences this inability to gain what he desires as "a total collapse."

6. (a) through (e) The definition of giftedness has broadened from a strict measure of intelligence to include a range of talents and personal attributes. "Most experts think that using a variety of formal and informal methods of identification is most effective," according to the editors of *Gifted Children Monthly* in their book, *Parents' Guide to Raising a Gifted Child* (Little, Brown, 1985). Given this new definition of giftedness, parents are apt to be in a better position than educators to identify a potentially gifted child. Other characteristics to keep an eye out for are curiosity and imagination, leadership, persistence, enthusiasm, ability in spatial relationships, planning ability, a wide range of interests, a preference for playing with older children, attention to detail, self-criticism (balanced by self-confidence), and, yes, good grades. If you feel your child excels in these various ways, you might talk to his or her school about testing for giftedness.

7. (e) That's right—fantasy is important work for a child, and yet parents are apt to interfere with their well-meaning praise, (c). Dr. Bettelheim says that kids need time to create this "secret garden." He explains that fantasy acts as a bridge between a child's inner and outer worlds, and has found that, if a person grows to adulthood without having learned to integrate the two, he or she may turn to drugs or psychoanalysis to reconcile them.

8. (c) The National Council of Teachers of Mathematics would be delighted if parents took the initiative of encouraging children to use calculators for everyday problems, such as tallying prices of meals in a restaurant (and the tip). The council cites an analysis of seventy-nine studies that show that "students who use calculators along with traditional instruction can improve their basic skills with paper and pencil." For a free pamphlet, *How to Be the Plus in Your Child's Mathematics Educa-*

tion, send a self-addressed, stamped business envelope to the council at 1906 Association Drive, Reston, Virginia 22091.

9. (a) Early-morning stomachaches are relatively common in the hours before school, according to a British study in the *Journal of Child Psychology and Psychiatry*. Psychosomatic tummy-aches affect about one child in ten, the researchers report, peaking at ages 5 or 6 among both boys and girls. Rarely is there an "organic," or purely physical, cause behind the pain—which isn't to say that the child's feelings about leaving home and going to school should be dismissed as unimportant.

10. (a) through (d) Patricia Lund Casserly of the Educational Testing Service reported that all of the above were likely to figure in the backgrounds of the 161 girls she studied.

11. (b) Teenage girls commonly think of themselves as having a weight problem when none exists. According to the study, reported in the *Journal of Child Psychology and Psychiatry* (March 1986), "although less than 4 percent were overweight as measured by standard tables, over 10 times this number considered themselves overweight." By the time the girls reached 18, more than half—55 percent—wanted to lose weight. As the researchers point out, an unwarranted weight loss can lead to illness.

12. (b) Eleven to twelve hours should do it. But children, like adults, vary in their sleep needs. Sleeping through the night will be a problem for most kids before they reach the age of 5. Some 70 percent will experience a period in which they awaken at least once a night, according to the New York Longitudinal Study of Temperament and Development.

13. (c) Skipping breakfast may drag down the performance of children who are already working to their capacity in school, according to Brian L. G. Morgan, Ph.D., a researcher in brain development.

14. (a) Surprised? That's the ringside observation of researcher Brian Sutton-Smith. Most amicable of all age/sex relationships was (d).

15. (c) Babies have more on the ball than adults have given them credit for. In fact, infants recently have been found to favor certain aspects of their environment—curved lines rather than straight, chromatic sounds rather than ugly ones, 3-D objects rather than flat ones, and complex patterns rather than simple ones.

16. (a) Young kids do well in counseling. According to James J. Muro and Don C. Dinkmeyer in *Counseling in the Elementary and Middle Schools* (William C. Brown, 1977), even when children can't or won't express themselves orally, their feelings are often obvious through their physical movements.

■ **SCORING**

Add the number of questions you got right, and see how you rank.

13–16: You are either a highly perceptive parent or a trivia hound.

9–12: You can consider yourself perceptive and well-informed.

4–8: Not bad, but you might consider browsing magazines as well as current books and professional journals on child development and psychology.

0–3: Well, you can console yourself with the fact that many of the opinions expressed in the "correct" answers are highly subject to the changing tides of child-rearing fashion. Today's commonly accepted bit of wisdom is apt to be tomorrow's quaint bromide.

HOW BALANCED IS YOUR CHILD'S DIET?

Balancing your family's diet is probably right up there on your list of priorities with balancing the family budget. There's no doubt about it—both call on all your skills as a juggler. Your bank balance tells you how you're doing on the financial front. It's a bit harder to tell with your family's diet.

For years we've been told that the key to good nutrition is eating a variety of foods from the four basic food groups every day. Who keeps score? But for the record that means four servings of a dairy product, two or more of meat or another protein food, four or more helpings of a fruit or vegetable, and four breads or starches. Not to mention a healthy dose of fiber-rich foods, and a skimpy amount of fatty ones.

But, according to most dietitians, *daily* balancing really isn't the crucial ingredient to healthy eating habits. Better, they say, to look at the broader picture, say a week or even a month of eating. Are your kids getting fresh fruits and vegetables on a regular basis? Are the meats they eat lean ones most of the time? Do you broil more often than fry? Steam rather than sauté? Most kids are okay if they *usually* eat well, say the experts. They don't have to be nutritionally perfect every single day.

So lighten up. Even though you'll want to keep a lid on too much fat and sugar, occasional "empty" calories aren't a problem if your child is of normal weight and not a budding couch potato. The average child between the ages of 4 and 10 needs about 1,700 to 2,400 calories a day for healthy growth. A child who is used to getting those calories through a wide variety of good foods is less likely to end up an adult battling cravings for fatty, salty, and sweet foods.

Our rather lighthearted quiz below has some solid nutritional information behind it. Taking it can tell you and your kids how close to or far from the ideal you are—and whether or not you could use a refresher course in healthy eating.

To take the quiz, read each of the following twenty questions and choose the answer that best fits your family's eating habits.

1. What's for breakfast at your house?
   (a) "What's breakfast?"
   (b) doughnuts, sweet rolls, or sugared cereal and milk
   (c) juice and whole grain toast, or cereal with fruit and milk, or hot cereal or soup, or leftovers from last night's dinner

2. Your kids think sugar-coated cereals
   (a) are essential to life and happiness.
   (b) are something you break down and buy occasionally.

(c) are found only on Saturday morning cartoon show commercials.

3. Lunch for your grade schooler
   (a) is almost always bologna on white bread.
   (b) usually features peanut butter.
   (c) most often includes tuna, sliced chicken, or turkey on whole wheat bread.

4. Dinner is prepared by Ronald or the Colonel
   (a) once a week.
   (b) a few times a month.
   (c) on rare occasions only.

5. Your kids eat white bread
   (a) every day.
   (b) only in bun form.
   (c) never, because they are only vaguely aware it exists.

6. Your kids believe hamburgers come
   (a) in Styrofoam packages.
   (b) out of a frying pan.
   (c) from under the broiler.

7. A family TV-time snack is
   (a) chips, twirls, and Technicolor puffs.
   (b) pretzels and "juice drinks."
   (c) a big bowl of unsalted air-popped popcorn.

8. Cake or cupcakes appear in your house
   (a) weekly.
   (b) monthly.
   (c) only wearing birthday candles.

9. To your kids, fruit is
   (a) punishment.
   (b) okay as a snack if there's nothing better.
   (c) their usual dessert or snack.

10. Your thirsty child will usually drink
    (a) anything as long as it's fizzy, sweet, and artificially colored.

(b) milk—you're thinking of buying a cow.

(c) water.

11. Cheese is

(a) smelly white stuff only grown-ups eat.

(b) found only on pizza and cheeseburgers.

(c) a standard at lunch, dinner, or snack time.

12. Potatoes, rice, or pasta appear on your table

(a) only if fried.

(b) a few times a week.

(c) at almost every meal, usually boiled or baked.

13. Green or yellow vegetables are

(a) better left at the supermarket.

(b) something you have to eat to get dessert.

(c) nice crunchy things, often finger foods.

14. Eggs are

(a) gross.

(b) okay if they're hidden in things like pancakes or French toast.

(c) part of breakfast or dinner once or twice a week.

15. Carrots and celery are

(a) stuff Bugs Bunny would walk a mile for, but not your kids.

(b) taken along on long car rides or picnics.

(c) packed in a bag in their lunch or put in a bowl on the dinner table.

16. You serve a meatless meal

(a) only if it's pizza without the pepperoni.

(b) as a once-in-a-while bean burrito.

(c) at least once or twice a week.

17. Fish is

(a) something you catch with a fishing pole and then throw back in.

(b) okay as long as it's breaded and fried.

(c) a nice change from meat.

18. Low-fat milk is
    (a) only for fat people on a diet.
    (b) what's at home; school has the real thing.
    (c) the real thing, if you're older than two.

19. You keep the salt
    (a) in the shaker on the table.
    (b) only on the stove.
    (c) in a cupboard for using on grease fires.

20. To your kids, chicken skin is
    (a) the best part of the bird.
    (b) a spicy, crispy treat.
    (c) gross—if you don't take it off, they will.

■ SCORING

Give yourself no points for each *a* answer, one point for each *b* answer, and two points for each *c* answer. If you scored between 0 and 20, your family's eating habits need an overhaul, ASAP. A score of 21 to 32 shows that you're making some good choices, but there's still plenty of room for improvement. If your score was between 33 and 40, give yourself a gold star and take the family out for a hot fudge sundae. But just this once.

■ ABOUT THE ANSWERS

You probably realized early on that the *a* answers were the poor nutritional choices, while the *c* answers were the approved ones. If you found yourself picking a lot of *b* answers, you may be relying too much on convenience or carry-out foods, or turning treats into everyday fare. Now that you know the right answers, how about giving this quiz to your kids to take and then working with them to improve their test scores?

IS YOUR CHILD ALLERGIC?

Jessica loves school—when she attends. Lately, Jessica wakes up many mornings with a stuffy nose, and her mother keeps her home from school. Although she is normally bright and attentive, Jessica's grades are beginning to fall.

Cameron starts his day with high energy, only to grow tired and cranky by noon, despite a good night's sleep. He sasses his Mom and Dad, and antagonizes his playmates.

Erin is a cherubic little girl with a sunny disposition—and a stomach that frequently acts up for no apparent reason.

Jessica, Cameron, and Erin—and thousands of children like them—are experiencing widely varying symptoms, all caused by the same problem: allergy. It's a disorder that takes on more disguises than any other health problem—and doesn't discriminate against age, race, or sex.

Children are particularly hard hit. One out of five has some form of allergy. And if you happen to have allergies yourself—in the form of asthma, hay fever, or dermatitis—your son or daughter has a fifty-fifty chance of developing one, too.

But that doesn't mean allergies are easy to detect. On the contrary, recognizing an allergy for what it is—and not some other illness—takes the investigative skills of a Bob Woodward and Carl Bernstein. Frustrated parents are often misled by symptoms that mimic a cold (sneezing and coughing), intestinal problems (colic, cramps, and vomiting), or skin disorders (hives, rashes, and swelling). Even wheezing or shortness of breath can be mistaken for other ailments.

Yet those are the most typical symptoms of allergy. If they're not present, however, it doesn't necessarily mean your child has escaped. That's because allergies can work in mysterious ways. So, if you're still suspicious, be on the lookout for certain symptoms. Ask yourself these questions:

▪ DOES YOUR CHILD HAVE ALLERGY "SHINERS"?

Dark, puffy circles under the eyes are common in children with allergies and are caused by the congestion of blood in the capillaries (tiny blood vessels) under the eyes, according to Warren Richards, M.D., head of allergy and clinical immunology at Children's Hospital of Los Angeles and clinical professor of pediatrics at the

University of Southern California. "Some 'shiners' take on a bluish discoloration and may suggest child abuse when none exists."

■ DOES YOUR CHILD EVER GIVE YOU THE ALLERGIC SALUTE?

"This is a gesture common to children with nasal allergy," continues Dr. Richards. "Itching prompts the child to repeatedly rub the nose, either up and down or sideways, and may cause nosebleeds. In time, this gesture can form a noticeable crease across the bridge of the nose."

■ DOES YOUR CHILD HAVE DIZZINESS AND RINGING IN THE EARS?

Allergy may cause swelling and fluid retention in the arteries and smaller blood vessels feeding the ear, causing dizziness and annoying inner-ear sounds.

■ DOES YOUR CHILD HAVE ECZEMA (ALLERGIC DERMATITIS)?

Children with allergies often have hypersensitive skin and are plagued by dryness, itching, redness, cracking, and watery discharges. Check your child's face, neck, inside creases of both elbows, hands, and knees, since those are the most common trouble spots.

■ DOES YOUR CHILD HAVE DIFFICULTY HEARING?

On-and-off hearing loss, popping in the ears, a feeling of fullness in the head, or ear pain may be due to an allergy that causes the lower end of the eustachian tubes to swell. If hearing loss occurs at a very young age, it may interfere with speech, according to the experts. Unfortunately, a school-age child with allergy-induced hearing loss may then be labeled as inattentive or not too bright.

■ DOES YOUR CHILD HAVE AN ITCHY THROAT?

Does your child clear his throat constantly, even in his sleep? Allergy may be causing postnasal drip, which in turn causes the trickle in the throat.

TRACKING DOWN THE CAUSE

Almost anything can trigger allergies: You name it, and somebody's kid is allergic to it. But certain foods and inhalants are more apt to bother your child than others. Milk, wheat, eggs, nuts, peanut butter, and citrus—the cornerstone of many children's diets—are particularly common allergens, especially in younger children. So are house dust, mold, pollen (from trees, weeds, and grass), and animal dander (particles clinging to fur and feathers).

Here's where the help of an allergist (a doctor board-certified in allergy and clinical immunology) comes in. To determine if, indeed, your child is allergic, and exactly to what, he will ask you dozens of questions about what your child eats, breathes, and touches. You can help your doctor diagnose your child's problem by answering his questions as thoroughly as possible. Here's a sample of what to expect:

■ HOW LONG DO SYMPTOMS LAST?

If sneezing and stuffiness last a few days, then disappear, your child probably has a cold. If sniffling and congestion linger, or occur more than six times a year, allergy is probably the cause.

■ ARE SYMPTOMS WORSE AT CERTAIN TIMES OF THE YEAR THAN OTHERS?

If your child's symptoms flare up in the spring and late summer or fall, then subside in winter, the child could be allergic to pollen, the powdery grains that burst from plants during the growing season. (Pollen is worse—and symptoms most severe—on a dry, windy day and better when it rains.) If your child feels worse during damp weather, he could be allergic to mold and mildew, which flourish during spring and fall, the wet seasons.

■ DOES YOUR CHILD SUFFER MORE DURING THE HEATING SEASON?

That suggests an allergy to fumes from burning fossil fuel, especially gas.

■ DO YOU HAVE PETS?

If your child's symptoms are worse when around animals—cats, dogs, gerbils, guinea pigs, hamsters, horses, or parakeets—dander could be the trigger. And don't forget that down comforters and feather pillows fall into this category, too.

■ DOES YOUR CHILD CRAVE CERTAIN FOODS—OR FEEL BETTER IF HE SKIPS A MEAL?

Ironically, either tendency may point to food allergy.

■ DID YOUR CHILD SUFFER COLIC AS AN INFANT?

Colic often precedes food allergy later in life.

Your answers to these questions can narrow down the list of likely suspects, but to help confirm the diagnosis, your doctor may want to conduct a battery of allergy tests.

WHAT ALLERGY TESTS CAN TELL YOU

Allergy tests don't come right out and tell you exactly what your child's allergic to. They simply detect the presence or absence of IgE antibodies or other immune substances that indicate the *likelihood* of an allergy.

To interpret the results, the doctor takes the child's actual experience into consideration, though. "For example, a child could have a positive reaction to dog dander [indicating allergy] yet suffer no nasal problems or other allergy symptoms when around the family dog," explains Edward W. Hein, M.D., chief of pediatric allergy at St. Christopher's Hospital for Children in Philadelphia. "It just means that the child is potentially allergic to dogs. In such a case, we wouldn't necessarily tell the parents to get rid of the dog, but we would note the reaction and suggest that the dog not sleep in the child's bedroom, to limit exposure."

Of course, if your child experiences symptoms around the dog *and* shows a positive reaction, he's probably allergic.

The most common type of allergy test is called the scratch test. Based on a hunch about what's making your child miserable, the doctor scratches a minute amount of a suspected allergen into the surface of the skin. If a red welt (called a wheal and flare reaction) appears, your child may be allergic.

Skin tests are not available for everything under the sun. For now, your doctor will only be able to test for possible allergy to foods, house dust, and mites (tiny insects that live in dust), tree, grass, and ragweed pollen, and mold and animal dander.

"Scratch tests give us a lot of good information," says Dr. Hein. "And most children tolerate them surprisingly well. In fact, parents are much more anxious about them than the kids themselves."

Blood tests are another possible way to identify an allergy. Called RASTs (radioallergosorbent tests), these disclose the same antibodies that scratch tests do, locating them in the blood instead of the skin.

"Blood tests are simpler to do and easier on the patients—you can test for several allergens with one sample," concedes Dr. Hein. "But the results take forty-eight hours, whereas the results of a skin test are obvious immediately. Blood tests are much more expensive than skin tests. And studies show that blood tests aren't as sensitive as skin tests. The RAST, for example, misses about twenty percent of the people who are allergic. That's bad news.

"Worse yet is that blood tests may give a false-positive result, indicating allergy when none exists," adds Dr. Hein. "Or the test may give a false-negative result. Here's why. The body first manufactures antibodies in the airway and gastrointestinal (G.I.) tract, which are then picked up and circulated by the blood. But if the antibodies linger in the nose, airway, or G.I. tract, the blood levels may remain normal. That happens in thirty or forty percent of people with hay fever or other respiratory allergy.

"It's possible that within five years blood tests may replace skin tests entirely," says Dr. Hein. "For now, the bugs need to be worked out, to make the test more sensitive and to lower the incidence of false-positive and false-negative results. But in situations where skin testing cannot be done, blood testing is a very good second choice."

Both skin and blood tests are especially limited in diagnosing food allergy. For one thing, foods may cause symptoms by a variety of mechanisms other than production of IgE antibodies (the presence of which, as we have seen, is revealed by skin or blood tests). And allergic reactions to food are often delayed, since it may take hours or days for the body to convert food into its allergenic particles.

"Since food allergies are not always picked up by skin or blood tests," says Dr. Hein, "any positive tests should be confirmed by a hypoallergenic diet." (That is, eliminate the suspected food or foods for three weeks, then reintroduce them one at a time to test for a reaction.)

OUTGROWING ALLERGIES

Even if the tests all indicate that your child is indeed allergic, here's a consoling thought from Dr. Hein. "My experience is that six out of ten allergic children tend to outgrow their symptoms. In fact, the earlier they develop an allergy, the more likely they are to outgrow it—usually around age six, or when they reach puberty."

As for asthma, adds Dr. Richards, 50 percent will feel better or be completely free of symptoms by puberty, too.

"That doesn't mean parents should sit back and do nothing, waiting for their children to outgrow the problem," Dr. Richards hastens to caution. "If a child is four years old and miserable, don't wait around—seek treatment."

Even if your child does outgrow his allergy symptoms, he may not be entirely home free. "Some kids may always retain a certain sensitivity when tested, yet still be able to tolerate the substance," says Dr. Hein. "In other words, a skin test may pick up allergic reactions, but the child may experience no discomfort when he eats or breathes the allergen."

Remember, if allergy becomes a lifelong condition, it's not the worst thing that can happen to your child. Most people can live quite comfortably with their allergies by learning to avoid those substances most likely to set them off and by following medical therapy.

IS YOUR BABY'S HEARING NORMAL?

More than 3 million American children have hearing loss. An estimated 1.3 million of these are under 3 years of age. You, the parents and grandparents, are usually the first to discover hearing loss in your babies, because you spend the most time with them. If at any time you suspect your baby has a hearing loss, discuss it with your doctor.

Your baby's hearing can be professionally tested at any age. Computerized hearing tests make it possible to screen newborns. Some babies are in a higher risk category for having hearing loss than others. If you circle any item *a* through *f* on this test, your child should have a hearing test as soon as possible, no later than at 3 months of age.

All children should have their hearing tested before they start school. This could reveal mild hearing losses that the parent or child cannot detect. Loss of hearing in one ear may also be determined in this way. Such a loss, although not obvious, may affect speech and language.

Hearing loss can even result from earwax or fluid in the ear. Many children with this type of hearing loss can have normal hearing restored through medical treatment or minor surgery.

In contrast to temporary hearing loss, some children have nerve deafness, which is permanent. Few, however, are totally deaf.

Most hearing-impaired children have some usable hearing. Early diagnosis, early fitting of hearing aids, and an early start on special educational programs can help maximize the child's existing hearing.

Use the following simple test to answer the question "Is Your Baby's Hearing Normal?"

PRESCHOOLERS' HEARING-LOSS RISK FACTORS AND TEST

Circle each item that applies:
(a) Family history of hearing loss, including brothers or sisters.
(b) History of illness in the mother during pregnancy, use of drugs during pregnancy, prolonged labor, or premature birth.
(c) Presence of other birth defects.
(d) Low birth weight or other physical problems at birth (e.g., jaundice).
(e) Child has had meningitis or scarlet fever.
(f) Child has chronic middle-ear infections and/or chronic upper respiratory allergies.

Giving each circled item 3 points, add score: _____

INFANTS (BIRTH THROUGH 12 MONTHS)	Almost always 0	Half the time 1	Infre- quently 2	Never 3
1. Nearby loud noise startles my baby and makes him/her move or even cry.				
2. Unexpected loud noise awakens my baby.				
3. My voice alone comforts or soothes my baby even when I do **not** pick him/her up.				
4. When my baby cannot see me, he/she turns eyes and head in the direction of my voice.				
5. My baby imitates noises.				

BABIES
(12 MONTHS THROUGH 3 YEARS)

1. My baby can point at familiar people or objects when asked.				
2. My **first** call gets a response.				
3. My child can imitate words. (If over 18 months, he/she can **use** a few words.)				
4. My child's speech and voice sound like other children's his/her age.				
5. My child listens to TV at a normal volume.				

TOTAL SCORE: Infant **or** Babies set plus risk factor = _____

■ SCORING

To calculate your baby's score, give 0 points for every time you check the "Almost always" column, 1 for every "Half the time," 2 for every "Infrequently," and 3 for every "Never." Add another 3 points for each item (a) through (f) that you circled above.

The American Academy of Otolaryngology—Head and Neck Surgery recommends the following:

0–5: Low risk of hearing loss. No immediate action is required.

6–12: Discuss the baby's hearing with your pediatrician, family physician, or ear physician.

13 and above: Strongly recommend that the child's hearing be evaluated by an ear, nose, and throat (ENT) specialist.

SIMPLE DO-IT-YOURSELF SCOLIOSIS CHECK

Children going through puberty sometimes feel as though their bodies have been taken over by strange forces. Certain things are growing, certain things are showing, and they wonder, "Am I normal?"

In most cases, physical development is right on track. But adolescence can bring a wayward curve in a part of the body they may not notice—the spine. We're talking about scoliosis, an abnormality that strikes roughly 5 percent of children starting as early as age 9, with girls seven times more likely than boys to get serious spinal curves.

Ideally, your child's spine should be straight when viewed from the back. But it's not uncommon for a slight, sideways S or C curve to develop. It's when this arch becomes more than slight that real problems begin.

"Out of every ten kids I see with a curve, two to three will actually have the disorder and need help," says Richard Martin, M.D., a pediatrician in Tucson, Arizona, and author of *A Parent's Guide to Childhood Symptoms* (St. Martin's Press, 1982). The problem is that you don't know whether the curve will stop after only a few degrees or take a serious turn for the worse. Later in life, a curve of 60 degrees or more can twist the rib cage and cause lung and heart impairment, a distorted appearance, back pain, and probably a relatively early death.

Recognizing the seriousness of scoliosis, the government, public schools, and national organizations have all jumped in to help.

Nineteen states have laws requiring public schools to set up screening programs for the disorder. The National Scoliosis Foundation recommends that schools annually screen children in grades 5 through 10, so that late-bloomers aren't overlooked. Unfortunately, while schools in just about every state screen voluntarily, not all of them cover kids throughout their growth years.

SPINE SIGNS

The screening given by school nurses, gym teachers, and doctors can also be done by the child-care provider who has your son's or daughter's best interest at heart—you. Your help may be especially important if your child's school doesn't begin screening by age 10 or doesn't do it annually, or if scoliosis runs in your family. According to Dr. Martin, if any adults in your family had it, your children are at higher risk. Also, if one child develops it, be sure to check your other children every year, possibly as early as age 6, he says.

You'll need 30 seconds and a chair, says Helen Horstmann, M.D., chief of pediatric orthopedics at the Medical College of Pennsylvania. Start by sitting down with your child standing in front of you. He or she should be bare from the waist up, facing away from you with feet together. Now, with knees locked, have him or her bend forward gently as if halfway attempting a toe-touch exercise. Arms should hang loosely, with the chin tucked toward the chest.

Examine the spine from the buttocks to the neck. The muscles on each side should hump slightly but evenly. There should not be more of a hump on one side. This bend-over technique is the best way to screen for scoliosis, according to the experts. But these five additional signs can be tip-offs to trouble, too.

- One shoulder blade is more prominent than the other.
- Hips and shoulders are uneven.
- When the child's arms are hanging, there is an unequal distance between the arms and body.
- The waist curves in more on one side.
- Clothing hangs unevenly. (Look at necklines and hemlines.)

If you suspect a problem is developing, take your child to your family physician. Depending on how much of a curve there is, your doctor will either keep close tabs on its progress or refer you for treatment to an orthopedic surgeon who specializes in scoliosis.

Children with moderate curves (20 to 40 degrees) are usually fitted with a lightweight, plastic, torso-hugging brace that's worn during their growing years. There is also an experimental night-time treatment that uses electrodes during sleep to stimulate the muscles near the spine gently. So far, this seems to be as effective as bracing. (Bracing and spinal stimulation stop the curves from increasing but don't improve them.) Serious curves (beyond 40 or 50 degrees) may require surgery. Scoliosis is easier to treat in the early stages, so the sooner you find the disorder, the better.

HOW FIT ARE YOUR KIDS?

Forget what it says in your child's report card under "Phys. Ed." George Allen's been keeping his own score. Says the legendary coach of the Washington Redskins and Los Angeles Rams, and former chairman of the President's Council on Physical Fitness and Sports, "If you're grading from A to F, where fitness is concerned, most would get an F.

"I've traveled around the world, and I can tell you that the kids in Europe and in the Orient are in better shape than American youngsters. The reason we should care is that our children are the future of our country. And if the youth of our country are lazy, out of shape, and don't eat properly, then all that America has stood for and accomplished is in jeopardy," says Allen.

A 1985 study conducted by the President's Council on Physical Fitness and Sports reveals that America's kids have *not* participated in this nation's fitness boom. At best they have shown virtually no improvement in fitness over the last ten years, and in some areas, test results have actually deteriorated.

According to the 1984 National Children and Youth Fitness

Study, "Youth of today carry substantially more body fat than their counterparts in the 1960s did." Only about half of America's next generation is getting enough physical activity to maintain sound cardiovascular health. And approximately half of today's youth do not meet the minimum requirements of vigorous physical activity year-round.

MOTIVATION AND SELF-DISCIPLINE

Clearly fitness has more to do with building a lifetime of good health habits than with keeping kids out of trouble or teaching them the finer points of volleyball. If we don't want to saddle our children—and our society—with unnecessary medical expenses later on, we have to start them on the road to health right now.

How do we do this? "It's all motivation," replies Allen. "Everything in life is motivation and self-discipline, trying to do better, to improve. If kids aren't physically fit, part of it is the parents' fault and part the schools' fault.

"The best coaches are the ones who set the pace themselves," Allen says, switching to pep-talk mode. "They work hard, and they have self-discipline. They work with the players, study hard, prepare the ball club to win. Parents can do that, too, by setting a good example. They should try to be in shape, work out, not be overweight, not smoke or drink, and not just sit around watching television. Parents should be working out and having the kids working out with them."

On the subject of school physical-fitness programs, Allen also has strong opinions—and a practical suggestion for improvement.

"The schools say they don't have the money to have physical-education classes five times a week, and that's partly true," says Allen. "But with gym classes only two or three times a week, you can't even begin to warm up.

"I think if I were running the schools, I would try to have a volunteer period every day where I got a bunch of boys and girls together to do something that would be fun that would also get them into shape, and I'd give the winners some kind of award."

ORGANIZED SPORTS AND FITNESS

What about organized sports? Will your child become physically fit just by playing sandlot baseball or touch football in the school playground? Actually, Allen says, sports are only part of the solution.

In Allen's opinion, "Kids have to work out at least three days a week (preferably five), a good hour every day, and not just playing right field, walking in and walking out. They have to do vigorous cardiovascular exercise under qualified supervision."

"Some of what kids do in organized sports does carry over into the rest of their lives. A good coach gets kids into shape. I played football, basketball, and ran track in school, and that physical activity carried over as a life-style for me, because I realized how much better it made me feel."

Today's children need an incentive to become healthier members of society. "The incentive," Allen says, "is to realize your potential."

Allen realizes that parents alone can do only so much to urge their kids on to accomplishment. "We are, and have been for two years, doing everything we can to get this idea going," he says. "We're running public-service announcements featuring the President of the United States. We're developing new fitness tests, with gold pins for kids who are physically fit. We're working on a model fitness program in Laguna Niguel, California, and we're going to build the United States Fitness Academy, with youth fitness its top priority."

HOW DO YOUR KIDS MEASURE UP?

If you want to know whether your children are building the fitness habits that will serve them well later in life, you can give them this simple test, developed by the President's Council on Physical Fitness and Sports.

Pull-Ups

- For boys: Go to your neighborhood playground or school gym and find a sturdy bar that is high enough off the ground that your child's feet clear the floor when he hangs from it. The child should grasp the bar with his palms facing away from his body. In smooth movements—jerky ones don't count—he should raise his chin above the bar as many times as possible. He must lower his body each time so that his arms are fully extended between pull-ups.

■ Passing grades: For ages 9 to 12, one pull-up; for ages 13 to 14, two pull-ups; and for ages 15 to 17, four pull-ups.

■ For girls: The recommended action is not a full pull-up, but what is called a flexed-arm hang. The bar should be the same height as the girl. The point of the test is for the child to grab the bar in the same position used by the boys—palms away from the body—and to hang from the bar, elbows flexed and chin above the bar, for as long as possible.

Passing grades: For all ages, the child should hold the flexed position for 5 seconds.

Sit-Ups

■ The child lies on his or her back with the knees bent, feet flat on the floor about 12 inches apart, and heels the same distance from the rear end. Hands go behind the neck, fingers interlaced. Sit up, moving forward until the elbows touch the knees. Do it as many times as possible.

Passing grades: For boys and girls of all ages, twenty sit-ups.

Recovery Index

■ You'll need a bench or stair step for this one, from 14 to 20 inches high, depending on how tall your child is.

It's a simple test. The child steps up with one foot, then the other, stands erect, then steps down with the first foot, then the other. Repeat.

Passing grades: For kids 9 to 12, 4 minutes without distress. Ages 13 to 17, 4 minutes without distress plus a score of fair or higher on the following index.

INDEX

After the 4-minute activity, the child rests for 1 minute. Then the child's pulse is taken for 30 seconds. (Just as you would with an adult, you locate the child's pulse on the side of the neck or on the thumb side of the wrist. Place the fingers, but not the thumb, over the pulse and count the beats in 15 seconds. Multiply the number by 4 to determine the number of beats per minute.) Take the pulse again after 2 minutes, and again after 3 minutes. Add the three pulse counts, then consult the following table:

PULSE COUNT	SCORE
199 or more	Poor
171–198	Fair
150–170	Good
133–149	Very good
132 or less	Excellent

This test should be administered to your child twice yearly. It's sometimes given at school. If you believe your child has unusual difficulty completing the test, and particularly if he or she has trouble with the recovery index test, please consult your physician, who is best qualified to evaluate the results.

IS YOUR PLAYGROUND SAFE?

The playground supervisor looked at her watch, sucked in her breath, and tightened her scarf. "Ten seconds," she predicted. "They'll be here in ten seconds." As if on cue, the double steel doors leading to the cafeteria exploded open, and 198 elementary school-children, who had been penned up all morning, charged out into the playground. The boys were in the lead. An even dozen headed out across the blacktopped basketball court to play soccer in an adjoining field. A group of girls scrambled after them to make sure that no soccer player put his dirty sneakers on their carefully chalked hopscotch squares.

The kids looked like what they were: a mixed bag of big, little, happy, sad, fast, and slow kids. But as the smallest of them wriggled his way to the top of the steel climber, there was one thing they were not—and that's safe. They weren't safe because, despite a computer-generated maintenance schedule that made sure their playground was kept in tip-top condition, some of the equipment was inherently unsafe. And the hard-packed dirt underneath was a killer.

Hard to believe? Not when you know the statistics. Over 207,000 children were treated for injuries on United States playgrounds in 1989. An earlier study by the Consumer Product Safety Commission (CPSC) revealed that 72 percent of the children injured on playgrounds were hurt in falls—falls in which a child hit a hard surface or hit the equipment on which he was climbing, or falls in which a child fell from one piece of equipment and hit another. And these were little kids. Four out of every five children injured were 10 years of age or younger.

Climbing apparatus (jungle gyms, chinning bars, etc.) are responsible for 42 percent of all playground injuries, estimates the Consumer Product Safety Commission—which makes sense, since children play on them more than any other piece of equipment. Swings account for 23 percent of the injuries and are second in popularity. Slides come in third; they're responsible for 16 percent of all injuries. Merry-go-rounds and seesaws are used significantly less than other equipment, but they still account for 11 percent of playground injuries.

How are our children getting hurt? They're slipping and losing their grip or their balance on monkey bars as they jump on and jump off, perform stunts, or swing from rung to rung. They're leaping from swings and falling, or standing too close and getting struck. They're falling from the sides, platforms, and ladders of slides as a result of walking up and down the slide, losing their grip or their balance, roughhousing, and just plain slipping. Occasionally they hit protruding bolts, strike the slide rim and edge, or just slip on the ladder and bang the steps.

If it sounds as though kids are getting battered at their local school or neighborhood playground, that just may be the case. But how can we prevent it? Short of sending out our kids in body armor or forbidding—fat chance!—their sneakered feet from leaving the ground, how can we keep our children safe?

CUSHIONED LANDINGS AND OTHER SAFETY MEASURES

One way is to cushion their landings, says Mike Gable, an administrator in the City of Pittsburgh's department of parks and recreation. That's exactly what Pittsburgh has begun to do. They're installing Greenpark Breakfall, a kind of synthetic cushioned mat made by Milwaukee's Donovan Flooring company, under anything with height—particularly monkey bars, slides, and swings. It may take them a while to get around to all the city's 150 or so parks and tot lots, says Gable, but they're definitely on the way.

Another way, says landscape architect Ira Berke, director of landscape construction for Chicago's Park District, is to provide close adult supervision. "If a school puts in playground equipment," says Berke, "then they have to provide the supervision." In a public park, parents have to assume the role.

"Don't get me wrong," Berke adds. "I agree that a resilient surface (like Breakfall) is nice. We're considering it now. But that's not the whole answer. Parental supervision is a part of it, too. When I used to take my daughter to the playground, I stood right there by any piece of equipment she was on. I didn't make it obvious," says Berke, "but I was there."

How else can we make our playgrounds safe? Go to your local playground and answer the following fifteen questions. The answers you get will tell you if there are safety problems where your kids play. To get action, start by reporting hazards to your city or town's municipal authority or—if it's a school playground—the school district's main office. You need to be certain your children are getting the safe playground environment they deserve.

1. Is there asphalt, concrete, or any other hard material under any playground equipment?

    If there is, say the Consumer Product people, move the equipment. Or install more resilient surfacing such as bark, wood chips, or shredded tires, outdoor rubber mats, or synthetic turf. These materials won't reduce the number of falls, but they may very well reduce the severity of injuries—an important point since nearly half of all injuries from falls will involve your child's head. A softer surface can mean the difference between a minor bruise and brain damage.

2. Are buildings, paths, gates, fences, and other play areas such as sandboxes at least eight feet away from the "use zone" of each piece of equipment?

    Your child needs enough room to exit slides, jump from swings, and spin off merry-go-rounds without worrying about running into other objects or people. If equipment is crowded together, says the CPSC, consider moving some pieces out of the more densely populated areas. Smoothly flowing traffic will eliminate collisions between your child and his buddies.

3. Are there any trees, shrubs, walls, or fences that can hamper supervision inside the area?

    Get rid of them. How will you—or a teacher, if it's a school playground—know when the local clown is standing on his head on top of the climber if you can't see him?

4. Is there a relatively impenetrable border such as a fence or trees around the entire playground?

    All playgrounds should be enclosed to prevent children from leaving the play area or running into a street, say the Consumer Product people.

5. Is all metal equipment painted or galvanized to prevent rust? Are all wood surfaces treated with a nontoxic substance to prevent the wood from rotting?

    And it's also a good idea, says the CPSC, to install or paint slip-resistant surfaces on the climbing and gripping components of all playground equipment.

6. Can children comfortably climb between horizontal bars?

    Your child may become trapped if the distance between bars is less than the height of his head, says the CPSC.

7. Is there any opening—a swinging exercise ring, for example—that is too small to allow your child to withdraw his head easily?

Obviously anything that can trap a child in any way should be removed. If there's no other way for a child to support his weight than his head or neck, for example, there's risk of strangulation.

8. Can you see anything that might catch at your child's clothing?

A piece of clothing caught on a bolt might be just enough to make your child lose his balance and fall.

9. Do you see any sharp points, corners, or edges? Any protrusions or projections? Any angle that might pinch or crush a finger?

Cover the exposed ends of bolts or tubing, get rid of pinch and crush possibilities, and slap brightly colored tape or paint on any protrusion to make it more visible.

10. Are the rungs on any climbing equipment small enough to be safely grasped by your child?

The bars on jungle gyms, monkey bars, domes, arch ladders, and other types of climbing equipment should be cylindrical and roughly 1⅝ inches in diameter, says the CPSC.

11. Is there a way out?

Sometimes it's easier to climb up than down. Make sure your child can climb either down or over to another piece of equipment for a descent that's as easy as his ascent.

12. Are any steps or rungs painted in bright, contrasting colors?

It's a good idea to highlight potentially dangerous climbs. Anything that can help your child perceive distances more accurately has got to make him safer.

13. Are any concrete footings exposed?

Cover them with earth or padding to prevent tripping and to protect your child in case of a fall, says the Consumer Product Safety Commission.

14. Are swings located away from other activities or equipment?

They should be. Otherwise your child may run into a moving swing as he chases a ball or does some other maneuver.

15. Do swings bump into one another?

Consider removing one or two swings from the swing set, suggests the CPSC. And what are the swing seats made of? Seats should be made of lightweight materials such as plastic, canvas, or rubber with smoothly finished or rounded edges. Add tire swings if you have the opportunity. Their safety record appears to be better than that of conventional swings.

THE NEXT STEP

So how does your playground measure up? Not so great? Then it's time for the next step.

- If it's a school playground, lodge a complaint with your school district superintendent, and send a copy of your letter to each member of the school board.
- If the playground is run by a municipality, complain to your town or city's department of parks and recreation with a carbon copy to each member of your city council or board of supervisors.
- Let your local newspaper know of your findings, too. You'll be surprised at how interested they'll be. They may even send a photographer to the playground to document the danger.

HOW TO CHOOSE THE RIGHT PEDIATRICIAN

Here are seven questions to ask your child's prospective doctor that he'd better get right, and four to ask yourself.

Your pediatrician may someday hold your child's life in his or her hands. So how do you go about finding just the right doctor? Someone you can trust to see you through medical crises, both large and small, throughout your youngster's childhood? It's one of the most important decisions a new parent has to make. With that in mind, we asked Robert A. Mendelson, M.D., a board-certified pediatrician, for his advice.

According to Dr. Mendelson, the time to find a pediatrician is before the baby is born. That may sound like putting the cart before the horse, but there's a good reason to decide on your child's doctor ahead of time. After all, you'll want to be prepared should the newborn need medical attention right away.

You can begin your search by getting a few good recommendations. "Start with those you admire both as people and as parents," advises Dr. Mendelson. "Ask them who their pediatrician is and, more important, if they would recommend that doctor for your family. Many people continue to see pediatricians they wouldn't recommend. It could be that the child is attached to the doctor. Or maybe they only see the pediatrician once or twice a year, and think it's too much trouble to switch."

Once you've got a recommendation, schedule a prenatal conference. Think of it as a job interview for the doctor. Although this practice is just now gaining wide popularity, Dr. Mendelson says he saw the need for the prenatal conference very early in his career.

Within 12 hours after a baby's birth, Dr. Mendelson sees his tiny patient for the first time. "We can pick up a lot during that first exam," he says. "Genital deformities, hip displacements, heart murmurs, eye abnormalities. It's hard for parents to hear from a stranger that something's wrong with their new baby. It's just as hard on the doctor to give bad news to someone he's never met before."

Plan to schedule prenatal conferences with several pediatricians. The actual number is hard to predict because your search will be over only when you have found the one you're comfortable with.

Schedule the conference when both parents can attend. "Even though the mother may be the primary caretaker, both parents need to feel they can deal effectively with their child's doctor in an emergency," says Dr. Mendelson. "Besides, with so many mothers working today, it's becoming more common for the father to bring in the child for office visits."

The doctor should use this opportunity to get the family's medical history—a process best done when each parent is there with information about him- or herself.

The cost of the conference will vary, so it's a good idea to ask about the fee when you call for an appointment. And don't wait until the last minute. Dr. Mendelson recommends beginning prenatal conferences during the seventh month of pregnancy to allow enough time to reflect on your choice.

Here's a list of questions to ask your prospective pediatrician and the answers you're looking for. Dr. Mendelson suggests that you bring a written list of questions with you. That way, you won't have to worry about forgetting what you meant to ask.

1. Are you available at night and on weekends?

Ask the doctor how you can reach him at these times, and find out what you should do in an emergency. "An appropriate response from the doctor would be 'Call me,' " says Dr. Mendelson. "An inappropriate answer is 'Go to the emergency room.'

"For one thing, you have no idea how much pediatric training the emergency room doctor has. For another, your pediatrician should always do a kind of 'triage,' or assessment of the situation, first, either in person or over the phone. He may want you to try treating the problem yourself before resorting to the emergency room. Fully half of the people who go to the emergency rooms could have been spared the time and expense if they had checked with their doctors first."

2. Who takes your calls if you're not available?

No doctor is available twenty-four hours a day, seven days a week. So it's best if your child's doctor is backed up by physicians who practice with him, particularly when a crisis arises. "Most parents are familiar with their child's medical history," says Dr. Mendelson, "but with a critical illness, quick access to office records can be crucial."

You also want to know if the replacement is equally qualified in treating children. In some cases, the stand-in doctor may be a family practitioner who has had much less training in pediatric care than your pediatrician.

3. Do you have a special time for nonurgent calls?

The doctor may have prescribed times when you can call him and when he returns calls. Those times should be convenient to your schedule. "I tell people to call whenever they want to," says Dr. Mendelson. "Then I return nonurgent calls at the end of the morning and the end of the afternoon."

4. When should I call you?

" 'Call me whenever you are worried about your child and it's something you can't handle' is the right answer," says Dr. Mendelson, "not 'when the child's temperature reaches a certain level or she goes into convulsions.' "

5. What are your fees?

Ask if the doctor has a written fee schedule to make comparison of fees between doctors easy. "Parents should know exactly what the doctor charges for services like well-baby visits and immunizations," says Dr. Mendelson."And they should feel comfortable asking about charges.

"You might also want to ask whether the doctor charges for telephone calls. Pediatricians spend more time than most doctors advising patients over the phone, and in some regions of the country it is customary to charge for that time."

6. What are your qualifications?

Dr. Mendelson recommends that your pediatrician be board-certified in pediatrics and be a member of the American Academy of Pediatrics.

7. Do you have children of your own?

"I don't recommend pediatricians who don't," says Dr. Mendelson. "It's much easier to empathize with a three A.M. call from someone who's been up all night caring for a child with the croup if you've been there yourself."

Of course, you may feel differently about this issue. That's why, in addition to the questions you ask the doctor, there are a few that you should ask yourself.

1. How important is this doctor's location?

You may want your pediatrician to be located close to your home, close to the school or day care your child will attend, or close to where you work.

2. Would I prefer a male or female pediatrician?

Although it probably won't matter to your baby, you may feel more comfortable dealing with either a man or a woman. If it's important to you, it should enter into your decision.

3. Is the doctor's age important to me?

Like gender, the age of the pediatrician is something to think about. Would you feel more confident with a younger doctor, who has been trained in the latest techniques, or would years of practical experience be more reassuring to you?

4. Do I like the doctor's personality?

The prenatal conference should give you a good idea what the doctor is like. What did you think of her? Did you like her manner? One way to avoid a personality clash between you and your pediatrician is by asking for the doctor's opinion on issues like breastfeeding, circumcision, working mothers, and after-hours calls. "The answers are not black and white, right or wrong," says Dr. Mendelson, "but the physician's approach in each case should be the same as yours."

PARENTS' RIGHTS:
DO YOU KNOW WHERE YOU STAND?

Many of us, as caring and responsible parents and grandparents, are quick to say we know all. But do we? In the innumerable medical situations that arise with children, are you prepared to stand firm on your rights as parents? Should your child have a chronic disease or a condition requiring hospitalization, do you know the barriers to full exercise of parental rights? Do you even know what those rights are?

Health care for children is unlike any other area of medicine in that the medical practitioner must deal with two consumers—the child and the parents. But doctors are trained to operate on a one-to-one basis—patient and practitioner. When parents are involved as a third party in that relationship, most doctors either ignore the parents during the examination of a child, and dictate rather than discuss treatment options with them, or they address themselves only to the parents and treat the child as an object to be studied. At one time or another, every parent with a sick child has left a doctor's office feeling confused or helpless, and there's absolutely no reason for this. The parents usually pay for the care *and* must make any necessary decisions regarding that care.

Truly informed decisions must come from a sound basis of knowledge. Here's a quiz to test *your* knowledge in a few areas. True or false:

1. A doctor can treat a child without the parents' permission in an emergency.

2. Parents have the right to refuse immunizations for their children.

3. In all cases teenagers must have their parents' permission to obtain medical care.

4. Any practitioner touching a child without parental consent is technically committing battery.

5. Even if a parent consents, a child can refuse to undergo treatment.

6. Parents do not have the right to decide when to remove life-supporting treatments, or "heroic measures," for terminally ill children.

7. A mentally ill minor child committed to an institution has no say in the completion of treatment and must await parental decision to be released.

8. Hospital policy can restrict or prevent visits to hospitalized children by parents.

9. The almost absolute right of parents requires that medical practitioners provide parents with all of the information they need to give informed consent for treatment of their child.

10. Parents do not have the right of access to their child's medical record.

■ **ANSWERS**

1. True.

Particularly if the child's injuries are life-threatening.

2. False.

Certain immunizations are mandatory in all states. In most cases parents can refuse immunizations for their children only on religious grounds or if an immunization would be medically harmful.

3. False.

Teenagers usually do not need their parents' permission in situations when it's necessary to protect the teenager's right to confidentiality (i.e., for contraception, treatment of sexually transmitted diseases, pregnancy, or drug and alcohol abuse).

4. True.

Battery is a criminal charge that can be applied when someone touches another person without permission in a potentially harmful way. (In different states, in different courts, the terms "assault," "battery," and "assault and battery" may be used interchangeably.) George Annas, an expert on health law, says in *The Rights of Patients: The Basic ACLU Guide to Patient Rights* (Carbondale: Southern Illinois University Press, 1989) that "since battery connotes an unauthorized touching, it is most applicable either when the doctor treats a patient without obtaining any consent (for example, a young child incapable of understanding), or when the doctor properly obtains consent for one type of operation but does another."

5. True.

Annas maintains that "little law . . . can be relied on to answer this question." Generally speaking, however, "a minor child who is competent to consent to treatment has the right to refuse the treatment."

6. False.

With one notable exception and within the guidelines established by state laws and case law, parents have the right to decide when to remove life-supporting treatments such as respirators. The courts have consistently supported parents' right to remove from life-support systems children who have been determined to be brain dead or in an irreversible coma. The one exception to this accepted parental authority involves seriously ill newborns; here, in general, the courts have supported a physician's decision to treat a seriously ill newborn without parental approval if the physician feels that the treatment will be clearly beneficial to the child.

7. True.

However, it is equally true that controversy surrounds parents' rights to make treatment decisions for mentally ill children. Mentally ill children who are committed to institutionally based treatments are not covered by the usual safeguards developed for involuntary commitments to institutions. Involuntarily committed patients have access to the court system to appeal the commitments. No such rights are generally given minors. Rather, in the case of minor children, such commitments are considered voluntary. (To be certain and specific, check to see what the age of majority is in your state for treatment of mental illness.)

8. False.

Parents have the legal right to be with their minor children at all times—in the doctor's office *or* the hospital. Annas says that "in general, if the law or the hospital requires the parent's consent for treatment of the child, the hospital cannot prevent or restrict parents from being with their children while in the hospital." He goes on to point out that the "only reasonable limits a hospital can probably place on parental visitation would involve actual interference with the hospital's ability to care for other patients (not the parents' child). . . . This would mean that parents, if they so desire, have the legal right to stay with their children during all tests and procedures, the induction of anesthesia, and to be present in the recovery room when the child regains consciousness."

9. True.

Parents can give informed consent only if the proposed treatment has been explained to them thoroughly, and all of the parents' questions have been answered to their satisfaction. In other words, practitioners are not legally permitted to ignore or dictate to parents, and parents—in the best interests of their children—can demand that their rights be recognized.

10. False.

If state law allows patients access to their medical records (and just over half of the states do), then parents have a similar right to their child's records. The only restrictions are those situations in which the child's right to confidentiality takes precedence over parents' rights. (A child's right to confidentiality varies from state to state, depending on the child's age.)

5. ARE YOU AN EMPOWERED MEDICAL CONSUMER?

Surveys report that up to 40 percent of the medical tests given by physicians are unnecessary. A study by the Equifax Corporation found that 98 percent of the hospital bills reviewed for the study had errors in them, and about 75 percent of those errors were in favor of the hospital. And finally, most consumers cannot read a prescription form, as important—and potent—as medications are.

Do you really know your medical rights? Can you discharge yourself from the hospital? Do you understand your health insurance? Are you using the right kind of specialist for your condition?

Testing your health IQ is more than just checking your pulse or knowing your personality type. It also means being savvy about the health-care system: how it works and what rights and recourse you have.

Studies show that informed and knowledgeable consumers get better health care. These same studies report that the medical outcomes of informed consumers are better than those who passively accept all that is put before them.

This chapter tests your medical consumerist IQ. The tests are unique. None will ever be given by your doctor, but they may be the most important self-care tests you ever take.

The tests in this chapter are designed to educate as much as surprise you. And when you have completed these examinations, you will be a far better-informed consumer than you were before you began.

YOUR MEDICAL RIGHTS: DO YOU REALLY KNOW THEM?

We're always talking about demanding our rights—but do we really know what our rights are? Do you know for sure which legal actions are under your control—and which are beyond it? Do you have a true handle on what kinds of moves you are empowered to take when it comes to your medical care, and especially the care when you are critically ill and perhaps even too ill to make decisions?

Test your knowledge of such things and see what your RQ—your Rights Quotient—really is. Take this quiz and see. It could mean the difference between first-class and low-class treatment, and it could help avoid family disruption and heartbreak.

The questions are based on current law, and in part on information from two sources sponsored by the American Civil Liberties Union: *The Rights of the Critically Ill* by John A. Robertson (New York: Bantam Books, 1983) and *The Rights of Patients: The Basic ACLU Guide to Patient Rights* by George J. Annas (Carbondale: Southern Illinois University Press, 1989). True or false:

1. There is a legal right to health care in the United States.

2. A doctor can lie to a patient about the seriousness of an illness if the doctor thinks it will spare the patient anxiety and grief.

3. A patient can override objections by the family and can demand to be told the nature of his or her illness.

4. A patient has the legal right to keep his or her illness a secret from the family.

5. The family has the legal right to stop treatment of a competent, critically ill family member, even if the patient wants it continued.

6. A cancer patient has a right to have his or her doctor prescribe or administer laetrile.

7. A competent adult can refuse medical care that could keep him or her alive.

8. If a doctor treats a patient against his or her will, in order to keep him or her alive, the patient can sue the doctor.

9. A patient can be thrown out of a hospital if he or she can't pay.

10. A doctor can (a) refuse to treat a patient who can't pay or (b) stop treating a patient who can't pay.

11. If, in an emergency, a person is brought to a hospital that does not have an emergency room, the hospital has an obligation to take in and care for the person anyway.

12. A hospital can prevent a patient from leaving.

13. A doctor must refer a patient to a specialist or seek a consultation if the patient requests it.

14. A doctor can refuse to continue to see a patient without first obtaining the services of another doctor for the patient.

15. A hospital patient has the right to refuse to be examined by medical students, interns, or residents.

■ ANSWERS

1. False.

Neither the Constitution nor federal or state law guarantees this right. There is no legal right to demand medical care.

2. False.

A doctor is obligated, under all circumstances, to tell a patient the diagnosis of his or her illness and its prognosis. If the doctor fails to do so, he or she can be sued for malpractice. If the patient has specifically expressed a desire to know the diagnosis and prognosis, and the doctor does not explain fully, it can be construed as a breach of contract. And, if the doctor keeps back information that ultimately obstructs crucial medical, financial, or personal decisions on the part of the patient, then the doctor could be held liable for the damages that result.

There are two instances where the doctor is off the legal hook: if the patient has specifically expressed a desire not to know, and if the doctor reasonably believes that bad news could do real harm to the patient (known as "therapeutic privilege").

3. True.

If the patient is competent, the family has no right to have information relevant to the person's medical condition withheld from him or her.

4. True.

A patient can ask that his or her condition be kept secret, and the doctor has to go along. That's part of what doctor-patient confidentiality is all about. Exceptions might include cases in which the release of information could protect others from contracting the disease or in which other harm could occur.

5. False.

If the ill person is competent (an important point) and also has the money to pay for treatments, the family has no legal power to stop it. The doctor's duty is to the ill person, not to family members. In terminal cases, the law is fuzzier. The patient has the right to treatment that will prolong life even a few days, but this right might not extend to include continued maximum treatment if he or she is in a comatose or unconscious state.

6. False.

Even in states where laetrile is legal, doctors aren't obligated to use it. Writes Robertson: "Since laetrile has not been shown to be effective, a doctor who refuses to prescribe it would not be violating his duty to provide the patient with effective medical care. If the patient objects, [he or she] is free to terminate the relationship and seek care elsewhere."

7. True.

According to some rulings, rejection of lifesaving treatment is protected by the constitutional guarantee of right of privacy. There would have to be some pretty good reason for interfering with this right.

8. True.

Despite a doctor's seeming good intentions or ethical concerns, he or she can be sued for battery, false imprisonment, or lack of informed consent. The doctor could even end up being responsible for the cost of the care. A patient can also get a court order, if necessary, to force a doctor to stop treatment on penalty of contempt of court.

9. False.

Once a person has been admitted and needs continued care, the hospital probably can't discharge him or her. The hospital could have the person transferred to another hospital, but only if the patient were in stable condition to be moved. If the patient is discharged because he or she can't pay, and then gets worse or incurs further damage, he or she could sue, claiming abandonment.

10. (a) True.
    (b) False.

Writes Robertson: "Although not obligated to begin treatment, once this is undertaken, [the doctor] is obligated to continue as long as the patient will benefit or [until] the patient withdraws." Otherwise, abandonment can be claimed, and a civil suit could follow. However, if the doctor has made clear at the start of treatment that ability to pay is a condition of continuing care, he or she can cut off treatment.

11. False.

In most states there is no legal obligation to do so, and a severely injured person could, within the law, be turned away. Some states have laws requiring hospitals to maintain emergency rooms. In these places, and in all situations where a hospital has an emergency room, that emergency room cannot turn away a person brought to it in an emergency state.

12. False.

If the person is of sound mind, he or she can leave at any time, and the hospital can't do a thing about it—or risk a suit for false imprisonment. And this applies even if the person hasn't paid his or her bill, or the bill for his or her child. A person may be asked to sign a "discharge against medical advice" form, but there is no legal obligation for the person to do so in order to leave the hospital.

13. True.

This is not a law, but good practice. It is also one of the American Medical Association's Principles of Medical Ethics. And if the doctor refuses a patient's request for a referral or consultation, and it turns out that the doctor's reassurance of proper treatment is wrong, a negligence suit is probably the patient's next (and probably successful) step.

14. False.

The only way a doctor-patient relationship ends is if (a) both parties agree to its end, (b) it is ended by the patient, (c) the doctor is no longer needed, or (d) the doctor has given reasonable notice. Otherwise, a case for abandonment can be made by the patient.

15. True.

Writes Annas: "All patients have a right to refuse to be examined by anyone in the hospital setting." In addition, fraud can be claimed if consent for an examination was given when a medical student was introduced as "doctor" to the patient, and the patient believed him or her to be a doctor.

WHERE ARE THE HAZARDS IN MODERN MEDICINE? DO YOU KNOW ENOUGH TO AVOID THEM?

Aside from the several celebrated cases of medical mismanagement that have made headlines, much of the ineptitude and misconduct in hospitals and physicians' offices nationwide goes unheralded. But more and more, consumer groups such as the People's Medical Society and other watchdog organizations are blowing away the smoke screen that has long obscured the real picture. Hospitals and standard medical practices are riddled with hazards, and only if you are forewarned and armed with knowledge can you hope to avoid those problem areas. Unfortunately, where medicine is concerned, the oft-repeated adage does not hold true: What you don't know *can* hurt you.

The following multiple choice quiz will test your knowledge of the hazards of modern medicine.

1. The approximate percentage of unnecessary surgery in the United States on an annual basis is
   (a) 8–10%   (b) 15–25%   (c) 35–45%   (d) 40–50%

2. According to a National Institutes of Health report, the percentage of unnecessary hysterectomies in the United States is estimated to be
   (a) 14%   (b) 20%   (c) 22%   (d) 32%

3. The estimated percentage of unnecessary cataract lens implant surgery, according to a government study, is
   (a) 8%   (b) 13%   (c) 18%   (d) 23%

4. The percentage of hospital patients who annually develop nosocomial (hospital-acquired) infections is
   (a) 2–5%   (b) 5–10%   (c) 10–12%   (d) 15–20%

5. The percentage of hospital patients with nosocomial pneumonia—the most common hospital-acquired infection—who die as a result of the infection is
   (a) 5%   (b) 10%   (c) 15%   (d) 20%

6. The number of deaths annually attributed to nosocomial infections is
   (a) 100,000   (b) 75,000   (c) 50,000   (d) 25,000

7. On any given day, the average number of medication errors committed in a typical hospital is
   (a) 25   (b) 175   (c) 250   (d) 360

8. The number of deaths annually attributed to anesthesia is
   (a) 10,000   (b) 12,500   (c) 18,000   (d) 22,000

9. The overall percentage of operating room deaths that have been attributed to errors in anesthesia, surgery, or both is
   (a) 60%   (b) 50%   (c) 40%   (d) 30%

10. The percentage of anesthesia-related mishaps that have been attributed to human error, according to national studies, is
    (a) 80%   (b) 60%   (c) 50%   (d) 30%

11. According to a published report, the percentage of X rays misread on an annual basis is
    (a) 5–10%   (b) 15–20%   (c) 20–40%   (d) 35–50%

12. The average number of people who develop cancer as a result of medical and dental X rays every year is
    (a) 17,000   (b) 51,000   (c) 67,000   (d) 78,000

13. The approximate percentage of people who suffer an unwanted side effect as a result of medication is
    (a) 40%   (b) 35%   (c) 20%   (d) 15%

14. The approximate annual percentage of physicians who are rendered incompetent to practice medicine because of alcohol, drug, or mental health impairment is
    (a) 1–5%   (b) 5–10%   (c) 10–15%   (d) 15–20%

15. The approximate percentage of illegible information found on hospital charts, according to a national study, is
    (a) 23%   (b) 37%   (c) 58%   (d) 66%

■ ANSWERS

1. (b) According to Robert G. Schneider, M.D., in *When to Say No to Surgery*, 15 to 25 percent of all surgery is unnecessary.

He estimated that of the between 20 and 25 million operations performed annually, some 3 to 6 million are unnecessary.

2. (c) According to a National Institute for Health Statistics report, 22 percent of all hysterectomies are unnecessary.

3. (d) The House Select Committee on Aging determined and reported that at least 23 percent of the 1 million cataract lens implants performed may not be necessary.

4. (b) According to a report by Milhap C. Nahata, Pharm.D., in *Drugs Intelligence and Clinical Pharmacy* (October 1985), between 5 and 10 percent of hospital patients acquire a nosocomial infection.

5. (c) According to a report in the *Western Journal of Medicine*, nosocomial pneumonia may be responsible for 15 percent of all hospital-associated deaths.

6. (a) According to another report by M.C. Nahata, there are no fewer than 100,000 nosocomial-related deaths annually in America.

7. (d) According to Neil M. Davis and Michael R. Cohen, in *Medication Errors*, in the average size hospital (between 250 and 350 beds) there will be 360 medication errors committed daily. Their formula takes into consideration the number of hospital patients, doses of medication, and the annual number of errors committed.

8. (a) Ellison C. Pierce, Jr., M.D., in an article entitled "Anesthesiology" appearing in the *Journal of the American Medical Association*, estimated that 10,000 people a year die as a result of inappropriate anesthesia administration.

9. (b) Victor W. Sidel, M.D., and Ruth Sidel, in their book *A Healthy State*, quote a physician as admitting that errors in judgment or technique concerning either the anesthesia or the surgery, or a combination of the two, contribute close to 50 percent of deaths in the operating room.

10. (a) According to William K. Hamilton, M.D., writing in *Anesthesia*, at least 80 percent of all anesthesia-related mishaps are due to human error.

11. (c) According to Leonard Berlin, M.D., in an article in the journal *Radiology*, 20 to 40 percent of all X rays are misread.

12. (d) According to John W. Gofman, M.D., and Egan O'Connor, in *X rays: Health Effects of Common Exams*, about 78,000 people a year get cancer from medical and dental X rays.

13. (a) According to published reports, about 40 percent of people undergoing medical care suffer side effects from the medication given them. This was reported by Martin Weitz in his book *Health Shock*.

14. (b) According to John Guinther, in *The Malpractitioners*, 5 to 10 percent of physicians are incompetent to practice medicine because of addictive, psychological, psychiatric, or other problems.

15. (c) According to Neil M. Davis and Michael R. Cohen, in a study on medication errors, they found that 58 percent of the information on hospital charts—and 80 percent of doctors' signatures—were illegible.

■ SCORING

15–13: Excellent. You obviously know where the dangers lurk and are prepared to guard against becoming a statistic.

12–10: Good. You've demonstrated that you're on the right track when it comes to identifying the danger zones of modern medical care.

9–7: Fair. Waste no time in becoming alert to the latest information on medical mistakes, ineptitude, and incompetence. Your life is at stake.

A TEST ABOUT UNNECESSARY TESTING

Over the years the People's Medical Society has had a lot to say about unnecessary testing. We've pointed out that millions of unnecessary tests and procedures are performed each year. Ultrasound tests of pregnant women, for instance, may not be needed or even useful as much as 30 percent of the time. Some hospitals routinely demand that each consumer be given a chest X ray upon admission, regardless of the consumer's ailment. The most unnecessarily repeated tests—a result of hospital policies—are blood tests and urinalysis.

Many physicians freely admit that too many medical tests are performed, and doctors regularly tell each other that "we would do well to use fewer tests now" (Jerome P. Kassirer, M.D., in the *New England Journal of Medicine*, June 1, 1989). Nonetheless, the overtesting continues, despite the recommendations to the contrary that roll out in the medical press. Apparently, some doctors still don't know—or don't care—about the hazards and the waste of unnecessary testing. And let's not forget the greed factor at work here.

And what about you? What's your Unnecessary Testing IQ? Here's a quick way to check yourself about medical tests and procedures and the way they are used (or abused) in our medical system. We've rounded up some of the more provocative studies on medical testing to form the following quiz. Grab your pencil and give it a try: You just may find that you're a sight more knowledgeable than many doctors out there. True or false:

1. Outmoded medical tests are abandoned when new, more precise high-tech tests come along.
2. Doctors know how much tests cost.
3. Four percent of hospital tests add up to half of a hospital's testing bill.
4. Walk-in clinic doctors increase the number of lab tests and X rays when they are offered a bonus to increase clinic revenues.
5. Tests performed in the privacy of a doctor's office are more accurate than those performed in large independent testing laboratories.

Now, let's see how your testing savvy stacks up.
1. False.

   In theory high-tech tests are designed to replace their

rougher, less precise cousins. In fact doctors are usually reluctant to let the old familiar tests go, so they use both tests. As Jerome P. Kassirer explains it: "Certainly not all duplicate testing is redundant, but many such tests are carried out merely to confirm a diagnosis that is virtually certain. Because of this, duplicate testing has been described as a 'belt and suspenders' approach—namely, one in which both are worn at the same time" (*New England Journal of Medicine*, June 1, 1989).

Just how common is the belt-and-suspenders approach to testing? A study published in the *Journal of the American Medical Association* (September 1, 1989) looked at pairs of diagnostic tests that consisted of one well-established diagnostic test and one new service that could largely substitute for the older one. The study's authors discovered that new technologies generally "complement" rather than replace older tests, even though the older test "often provides the same information." The "gradual accretion of technology," as the authors term it, contributes to the increasing cost of medical care.

2. False.

Physicians tend to think diagnostic tests are less expensive than they actually are. It's just one more factor that encourages them to overorder tests.

The latest study to confirm this appeared in the May 24, 1990, issue of the *New England Journal of Medicine*. In the study Indiana University School of Medicine physicians working at an Indianapolis health center were quizzed about the costs of tests. Their responses were wide of the mark "by an average of *more than 40 percent*," say the study's authors [italics ours]. Doctors generally don't know, because they themselves usually don't do the tests, decide on the charges, or do the billing.

On the positive side, the study showed that doctors had second thoughts about the necessity of tests when they were made aware of the costs. Those physicians who were shown test prices on a computer screen ordered 14 percent fewer tests—and generated bills approximately 13 percent lower—than physicians who did not see the price.

The study's authors predicted a $25,000 annual savings for consumers and insurers if all physicians at the health center were shown test prices. Imagine the savings to the consumer if all doctors in the United States were made aware of actual costs of medical tests. Unfortunately, the study also showed that, once doctors were no longer shown the cost of tests each time the tests were ordered, the number of tests drifted upward again. As they say, out of sight, out of mind.

3. True.

A fraction—only 4 percent—of tests performed are responsible for half of a hospital's testing bills, at least at Brigham and Woman's Hospital in Boston. That's where researchers examined 32,206 medical tests performed on 1,000 randomly selected patients (an average of 32 tests a patient!) in 1982. The total cost of the tests: $676,114. While the high-cost procedures—tests costing more than $100—were 4 percent of all tests performed, they accounted for 50 percent of the total testing costs incurred by the hospital and its physicians.

The study suggests that, if consumers and insurers wish to encourage cost-effective use of diagnostic testing, then attention should be directed first at reducing the unnecessary use of high-cost tests.

4. True.

For decades American business has used the bonus as a simple but effective means of increasing company sales. Considering the increasing commercialization of modern medicine, it's no surprise that bonuses and incentive plans have wended their way into the hearts of profit-making medical clinics.

A small study reported in the April 12, 1990, *New England Journal of Medicine* examined fifteen doctors' patterns of diagnostic testing at a Boston-area chain of walk-in medical clinics, which had just begun an incentive program. According to the researchers, "Physicians increased the number of laboratory tests performed per patient visit by 23 percent and the number of X-ray films per visit by 16 percent. The total charges per month, adjusted for inflation, grew 20 percent, mostly as a result of a 12 percent increase in the average number of patient visits per month."

Although the researchers said they found little evidence of "gross overtreatment" (a *small* comfort for the consumer subjected to unnecessary testing), and although the researchers noted that "extrapolation of our findings may not be warranted" because they examined only fifteen physicians, their research still raises serious concerns about the use of incentive plans in a medical setting.

5. False.

There's no guarantee that tests performed in a doctor's office are more accurate than those performed in large independent testing laboratories. Thanks to the advent of new, affordable technology, physicians are now able to set up small but profitable testing laboratories in their own offices. Unfortunately, some of these in-office labs are poorly run, staffed with employees who have no education or training to perform lab analysis, and lacking any sort of quality control program to see that tests are done right. The accuracy of tests performed in such sloppy environments is questionable.

This is not to say that commercial labs are models of precision and accuracy. For instance, in 1989 the *Journal of the American Medical Association* published a report that caused a reevaluation of quality standards for Pap smears. Ten to 20 percent of routine Pap tests were inadequate in some way, according to the report, and the most common causes were lack of information, inadequate cervical cell samples, and poor quality control measures. Additionally, some "Pap mills" were paving the way for inaccuracy by pushing technicians to process 200 to 300 Pap smears a day. (The recommended limit is *90 screenings per technician per day.*)

Concern about lack of consistency and accuracy in test results led Congress to pass the Clinical Laboratory Improvement Amendments of 1988. The legislation is designed to apply quality control standards to approximately 300,000 labs, both large and small, in the doctor's office and outside it, with some requirements taking effect in 1991 and others postponed way beyond the official start-up date.

DOES YOUR DOCTOR TREAT YOU WITH THE RESPECT YOU DESERVE?

How respectful is your doctor of your rights and dignity? How willing to impart vital information to you and how concerned about the cost of care? Is your doctor including you in the decision-making process in matters affecting *your* health, *your* body? Is he or she telling you everything you need to know in order for you to have an equal voice in your own health decisions?

The light of consumerism is shining on nearly every service we now receive: Automobile service shops not only give you an estimate before the job is done, but most call if the necessary work is going to exceed the estimated price. If you are buying a house, you receive a statement that explains what the monthly payments will be once you have moved in, as well as the costs associated with closing the deal. But there's one important exception—the medical world. Most doctors and hospitals continue to operate in a sort of medical Albania. They expect to be autocrats where *your* health is concerned, controlling all the lines of communication and making all the important decisions.

You can change all that, but first you need a code of straightforward and consumer-oriented standards. And second, you must decide what side of the line *your* doctor stands: your side or across the border in Albania. The quiz questions below provide the framework for this code. Take the quiz and grade your doctor on his or her willingness to embrace the medical consumerist movement.

■ SCORING

5 points if your doctor *always* does
4 points if your doctor does *most of the time*

3 points if your doctor *sometimes* does
2 points if your doctor *rarely* does
1 point if your doctor *never* does

1. Does your doctor post or provide a printed schedule of his or her fees for office visits, procedures, testing, and surgery?

2. Does your doctor provide itemized bills?

3. If you are on Medicare, Medicaid, or another form of insurance, does your doctor indicate that such coverage may not cover the total cost of services performed?

4. Does your doctor offer a flexible payment schedule?

5. Does your doctor provide certain hours each week when he or she is available for nonemergency telephone consultation?

6. Does your doctor promptly report test results to you and return phone calls?

7. Does your doctor schedule appointments to allow the necessary time to see you with minimal waiting?

8. Does your doctor allow you to bring a friend or relative into the examining room with you?

9. Does your doctor spend enough time with you?

10. Does your doctor facilitate your getting your medical and hospital records?

11. Does your doctor provide you with copies of your test results?

12. Does your doctor let you know your prognosis, including whether your condition is terminal or will cause disability or pain?

13. Does your doctor explain why he or she believes further diagnostic activity or treatment is necessary?

14. Does your doctor discuss diagnostic, treatment, and medication options for your particular problem with you?

15. Does your doctor describe in understandable terms the risk of each alternative, the chances of success, the possibility of pain,

the effect on your functioning, the number of visits each would entail, and the cost of each alternative?

16. Does your doctor discuss any possible negative side effects of the tests, treatments, and/or medications recommended?

17. Does your doctor describe his or her qualifications to perform the proposed diagnostic measures or treatments?

18. Does your doctor provide information about the prevention of your particular problem's recurrence in the future?

19. Does your doctor let you know of organizations, support groups, and medical and lay publications that can assist you in understanding, monitoring, and treating your problem?

20. Does your doctor wait to proceed until you are satisfied that you understand the benefits and risks of each alternative and have agreed on a particular course of action?

100–90: Congratulations! This doctor is right on track and running his or her business the way you, the customer, have every right to expect.

89–80: This doctor appears to be doing a pretty good job, but there's room for some improvement here. In not every case is he or she discussing and designing ways for both of you to work together to maintain and improve your good health. With a little tutoring, this doctor has a very good chance of pulling up his or her grade.

79–70: You may expect to be treated honestly and forthrightly by this doctor, but he or she is meeting you only halfway. The question you need to ask yourself, a wise consumer, is: Is average good enough where your health is concerned? If not, and if the doctor doesn't change and change soon, it's time to shop around.

69–60: Start calling around. This doctor's hanging on by slender threads. As the medical consumerist movement continues to grow, you won't be the only one seeking other doctors' services.

59 and below: The lights are already out in this doctor's practice. Not only is this doctor completely in the dark about emerging medical consumerism, but he or she is leaving you in the dark, too, about your health and appropriate medical services.

DO YOU KNOW WHICH MEDICAL SPECIALIST DOES WHAT—AND WHERE?

The medical world keeps coming up with new medical specialties as quickly as they discover new things wrong with you. And it's important for you to know just what the specialties of the specialists are. Who does what and where? Why should you be billed for the opinion of an ear specialist when the problem is in your foot? Granted, such a conniving consult doesn't happen very often, but it happens often enough. If it happens to you once, that's once too often. How can you protect yourself from such fraud? Know the physician specialties from head to toe. Here's a quiz to see how far you get. We've made it simpler for you by listing the choices of specialists— you just have to match the number on the drawing to the correct specialist from the list. (Figure 3, page 168.)

neurosurgeon
plastic surgeon
psychiatrist
gynecologist
urologist
thoracic surgeon
proctologist
ophthalmologist
nephrologist

allergist
endocrinologist
orthopedist
cardiologist
otorhinolaryngologist
neurologist
gastroenterologist
obstetrician

■ ANSWERS

1. Plastic surgeon.

Restores and rebuilds body parts damaged or destroyed by accident or disease; corrects or improves structures that don't live up to the individual's or society's standards. The indicator in the illustration points to the face and head because plastic surgeons do much of their work in this area: rhytidectomy (face-lift); blepharoplasty (eyelid surgery); rhinoplasty (nose job); otoplasty (change of shape or display of ears); hair transplant; dermabrasion and chemical peel (removal of skin layers

Figure 3

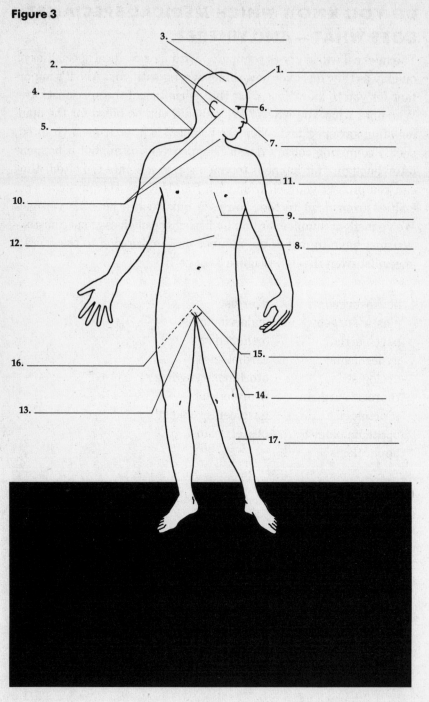

to make wrinkles and scars fade or disappear); mentoplasty (restructuring of jaws and chins); skin grafts. Of course, plastic surgeons also rework other problems in other parts of the body, breast enlargement or reduction (mammoplasty) and "tummy tucks" among them.

2. Otorhinolaryngologist.

This is the ENT—ear, nose, and throat—specialist who explores problems and treats disease in those three interrelated portions of the body.

3. Psychiatrist.

The psychiatrist is involved in examining, treating, and preventing mental illness. (Don't confuse this specialist with the nonphysician psychologist.) A psychiatrist's repertoire may include everything from the noninvasive (psychoanalysis) to the pharmaceutical; his or her observations and diagnoses may determine that the problem may be relieved only through surgery.

4. Neurologist.

This doctor is involved with the diagnosis and treatment of nervous system disorders.

5. Neurosurgeon.

Surgery on the nervous system (the brain, spinal cord, and nerves) is this doctor's field of expertise.

6. Ophthalmologist.

The ophthalmologist diagnoses and treats diseases of and injuries to the eye. He or she can perform cataract removals and retina reattachments, among other operations.

7. Allergist.

As the name implies, this specialist is involved in the diagnosis and treatment of allergies. Allergists often subspecialize in a single form of allergy. The indicator in the illustration points to the nose as the allergist's primary area of expertise, because hay fever and other conditions caused by airborne substances do make up a lot of his or her practice. However, this specialist also examines and treats asthma cases and skin problems all over the body (for example, hives and contact dermatitis).

8. Nephrologist.

Deals with diseases of the kidney.

9. Cardiologist.

This specialist diagnoses and treats heart disease. He or she may perform cardiac catheterization (snaking a catheter through a vein or artery and on into the heart to take certain measurements and examine heart structures) and pacemaker implantation. The cardiologist may also oversee the administration of stress tests, among other procedures.

10. Endocrinologist.

This specialist's field includes the diagnosis and treatment of disorders of the endocrine glands. Although the indicator in the illustration points to the general head and neck area—where the pituitary, thyroid, and parathyroids are—endocrine glands are located in other parts of the body: the ovaries, testes, thymus, and the pancreas's islets of Langerhans. (The islets of Langerhans secrete insulin, which explains why endocrinologists are involved in the treatment of diabetes.) Endocrinologists also treat problems of obesity.

11. Thoracic surgeon.

This doctor performs operations on the heart and major vessels and the lungs. Surgical procedures on the trachea and esophagus also fall within the scope of this specialty, as do operations to repair hiatal hernias.

12. Gastroenterologist.

The specialty here is the diagnosis and treatment of problems of the stomach and intestines, the G.I. tract.

13. Urologist.

Diagnoses and treats diseases of the urinary system, as well as the organs of reproduction in men, such as the prostate.

14. Gynecologist.

Diagnoses and treats problems associated with the female reproductive organs.

15. Obstetrician.

The specialty is in the medical aspects of and intervention in pregnancy and labor.

16. Proctologist.

This physician deals with diseases of the anus, rectum, and colon.

17. Orthopedist.

This doctor's domain includes the treatment and correction, usually surgically, of deformities or damage to the musculoskeletal system. Although the indicator in the illustration points to the leg area, orthopedic surgeons (sometimes referred to as orthopods) work on bone, muscle, and ligament problems all over the body.

DO YOU KNOW YOUR HOSPITAL RIGHTS?

How well do you know your rights when you're admitted to the hospital? Believe it or not, you do have rights when you're a hospital patient, and you don't need to sign your life away just to receive treatment.

Some of these rights are mandated by state legislation or health department regulations and are part of hospital licensure requirements. Others were written by the hospital industry and are promoted by its trade association, the American Hospital Association. Still others are the result of consumers learning more about the medical care delivery system and demanding that their rights be protected.

Test your knowledge of hospital patients' rights so that when the time comes you won't be guessing about your rights—you'll know them. True or false:

1. A hospital patient has the right to receive all pertinent information concerning his or her diagnosis, treatment, and prognosis presented in language that any layperson can understand.

2. A hospital patient has the right to receive all the information necessary prior to giving consent for any medical treatment or procedure.

3. When a hospital patient signs a consent form, he or she is relieving the hospital and doctor of all liability involving his or her care.

4. A hospital patient has the right to modify or change the standard hospital consent form in order to limit the number of procedures that may be performed.

5. A hospital patient has no right to refuse treatment once the doctor has selected the preferred course of treatment.

6. The hospital is under no obligation to advise a patient of the consequences of refusing treatment.

7. A hospital has an obligation to provide a patient with information about all medically significant alternative treatments if the patient makes such a request.

8. A hospital has the right to demand payment before a patient is discharged.

9. A patient has the right to be informed if his or her treatment is part of a human research experiment and has the right to refuse to participate in such research projects.

10. A patient has the right to expect that all communication and correspondence concerning his or her treatment be kept confidential.

11. The hospital is under no obligation to send the patient a copy of his or her hospital bill if it is being paid by an insurance company.

12. The hospital is not required to provide a patient with the names of other physicians who may be involved in providing care.

13. A hospital patient has the right to know if an economic relationship exists between his or her physician and the hospital, such

as the physician being an investor in the laboratory that has a contract with the hospital.

14. A hospital always has the right to transfer a patient for medical reasons.

15. A patient has the right to sign out of the hospital "against medical advice" (what the medicos call AMA) at any time during his or her stay.

16. Hospitals have the right to bring in a consulting physician to examine a patient and assist in his or her care, without the patient's prior permission.

17. A hospital patient always has the right to expect considerate and respectful care.

18. Hospital patients have the right to be informed in advance of all appointments and treatments that have been scheduled for them.

19. Hospitals are under no obligation to provide patients with information on hospital policies and procedures relative to patients' rights.

20. Hospital patients have the right to expect that hospitals will make every effort to respond to all reasonable requests for services.

■ **ANSWERS**

1. True.

   Most laws regulating medicine mandate this. And item 2 of the American Hospital Association's (AHA) Patient's Bill of Rights states that you have the right to receive complete, current information concerning your diagnosis, treatment, and prognosis. Further, all this must be presented in language that you can be reasonably expected to understand.

2. True.

   The legal informed-consent doctrine requires that you be given all pertinent information before making a valid decision.

(The only exception would be in the case of an emergency, in which you would be in no condition to make such a decision.) Informed consent is the most important legal doctrine in the physician-patient relationship, and has been so stated by the courts. The AHA Patient's Bill of Rights also supports your right to be fully informed.

3. False.

You cannot be forced to waive your rights to sue either a physician or a hospital. The courts have found that you are at a great disadvantage when it comes to bargaining with a hospital and, therefore, would feel compelled to sign any agreement presented by the hospital. Requiring this waiver of liability before providing treatment has been held to be illegal.

4. True.

You may need to sign these forms, but you can also make modifications. When you are given the blanket consent form, read it carefully and, if necessary, revise it. You have the right to insist that you will not agree to the procedure unless Dr. X performs it. The form is a contract that's subject to revision, and you have the right to revise it.

5. False.

You have the right to say no or stop treatment at any time. The doctor and hospital are legally bound not to treat you against your will. You also do not need to justify your reasons for stopping or refusing treatment.

6. False.

If you refuse treatment, the hospital is obligated to advise you of the consequences of your act. You will probably be asked to sign a document that explains what could happen to you and releases the hospital from liability.

7. True.

The doctrine of informed consent requires that you be told what the hospital intends to do, what is involved, what the risks are, and what, if any, are the alternatives. The description of the alternatives must include the types of treatments or procedures as well as the risks and benefits of the alternatives.

8. False.

Don't let a doctor, nurse, or hospital bureaucrat tell you that you must pay your bill before being discharged. You have an absolute right to be discharged at any time, even though you haven't paid one penny of your bill. Anyone who tries to hold you against your will is guilty of false imprisonment.

9. True.

You are never under any obligation to participate in any research, and you are not obligated to justify your refusal. The legal right for this goes back to World War II, when horrible medical experiments were perpetrated in Nazi concentration camps. If you are the uninformed victim of an experiment—and damages result from it—you have the right to file a medical malpractice suit against the doctor.

10. True.

You have the right to expect that all communication involving your care be kept confidential. This is both an ethical and a legal obligation. Historically, it goes back to the Hippocratic Oath, and more recently it has become part of state licensing laws. The AHA Patient's Bill of Rights also recognizes the obligation to protect patient confidentiality.

11. False.

The AHA Patient's Bill of Rights gives you the right to receive and examine a copy of your hospital bill. You must also be told how to obtain an itemized bill if you are given only a summary bill upon your discharge.

12. False.

The right to know the names of all the physicians who may be involved in your care is found in the doctrine of informed consent. In addition, this right is recognized by the AHA Patient's Bill of Rights.

13. True.

At least four states have passed laws that require doctors to tell you if they have any financial interest in a health care or other related facility. The AHA Patient's Bill of Rights also requires that any hospital financial interests be disclosed to you.

14. False.

Under regulations adopted by Congress in 1986, there are very specific instances when patients may be transferred. You must be informed of the pending transfer and must agree to it. In addition, the receiving hospital must have the space and personnel to treat you. This right is also recognized by the AHA Patient's Bill of Rights.

15. True.

You may leave a hospital at any time during your stay. The only exception would be if you were a danger to yourself or others. The hospital may ask you to sign a form that states you are leaving AMA (against medical advice). However, you are under no obligation to sign this document. If the hospital refuses to release you, it could be cited for false imprisonment.

16. False.

The doctrines of confidentiality and privacy prevent hospitals from bringing in consultants without your permission. This also applies to you even if you are admitted to a teaching hospital and your case is being considered for grand rounds. The hospital is obligated to obtain your consent. The AHA Patient's Bill of Rights also recognizes your right to approve any consultant assigned to your case.

17. True.

Your right to considerate and respectful care is recognized by the Joint Commission on the Accreditation of Healthcare Organizations and is part of its accreditation manual. The AHA Patient's Bill of Rights recognizes this obligation, too, which has also been incorporated into some state licensing laws.

18. True.

The doctrine of informed consent requires that hospitals tell you when appointments and treatments have been scheduled. You are also entitled to know who is responsible for scheduling and providing the treatments. The doctrine of informed consent exists to (a) promote the consumer's self-determination and (b) ensure that his or her decision-making is rational.

19. False.

According to the AHA Patient's Bill of Rights, you are entitled to receive a written copy of your rights. These rights should also be posted in every patient's room. While this requirement may not be a legal right, it is a human right nonetheless.

20. True.

According to the AHA Patient's Bill of Rights, you are entitled to expect that the hospital, within its capacity, will make a reasonable response to your requests for services. Once again, this may not be a legal right, but it is a human right.

■ SCORING

20–16: Excellent. You are well informed and educated on the subject of hospital patients' rights. You'll never be the patient left in the hall passively waiting while half the hospital goes on coffee break.

15–11: Good. But your ignorance of nearly half of the rights *you're* entitled to puts you at high risk of being pushed around by hospital staffers unresponsive to the patient's true needs and rights.

Below 11: Watch out! You just may find yourself at the mercy of probing doctors whose faces and names are unfamiliar and shuffled around from department to department and consult to consult (or worse). Get in the know—you *do* have a say-so.

DOES YOUR HOSPITAL BILL PASS THIS TEST?

National auditing firms have discovered that more than 90 percent of hospital bills contain errors, and those errors are usually in favor of the hospital. This means that you or your insurance company is paying for services not provided, or worse yet, paying twice for the same service. To add insult to injury, you practically have to beg the billing office for a copy of your statement, and then must cope with a myriad of undecipherable figures.

Hospital billing statements must have been designed by spies, because the coding system that is used is harder to crack than the Enigma machine of World War II. This usually results in frustration and anger at not being able to figure out quickly and easily what you were charged or what you owe. But you can even the odds by learning how to examine your hospital bill and knowing where to check for the most common errors.

The following checklist will show you how to spot those areas where most hospital billing errors occur. (Use the sample bill and follow the numbered questions, which correspond to the numbered portions of the bill.) The next time you find yourself stymied and/or outraged by a hospital bill, see if it can pass this test. And if not, immediately contact the hospital billing office and demand a more explicit statement or an audit.

1. Does the patient identification line or box contain the correct name and account number? (Some hospitals use your Social Security number as an account number, so check it closely—is it accurate?)

2. Are the admission and discharge dates correct? (You don't want to be billed for services if you were discharged before the next billing day.)

3. Is the name of the insurance company entered on the correct line or box?

4. Is the insurance group number correct? (A faulty number here could put you in the wrong group and delay your claim.)

5. Is the insurance policy number correct? (The wrong number here could lead to a rejection of your claim.)

6. Does the "bill to" line or box contain the correct name and address of the person who is responsible for paying the bill?

PATIENT ACCOUNT STATEMENT

GENERAL INFORMATION

PATIENT'S NAME	ACCOUNT NO.	BIRTH DATE	ADMISSION DATE	DISCHARGE DATE	STATEMENT DATE
JOHN R. DOE ①	123456	3-5-55	12-29-89 ②	1-20-90	1-27-90

PRIMARY INSURANCE CO.	GROUP NO.	POLICY NUMBER
HEALTH AMERICA/MAXICARE ③	584003 ④	185329253 ⑤

BILL TO / MAKE CHECK PAYABLE TO / AMOUNT OF YOUR PAYMENT

BILL TO	MAKE CHECK PAYABLE TO	AMOUNT OF YOUR PAYMENT
MARY ANN DOE ⑥ 987 10TH STREET TOPEKA, KS 66217	JEFFERSON HOSPITAL PO BOX 1990 J TOPEKA, KS 66201	$3526.80 ⑭

IMPORTANT: TO ENSURE PROPER CREDIT, PLEASE DETACH AND RETURN THE TOP PORTION OF THIS STATEMENT WITH YOUR PAYMENT

GENERAL INFORMATION

PATIENT'S NAME	ACCOUNT NO.	STATEMENT DATE	ADMISSION DATE	DISCHARGE DATE	PAGE NO.
JOHN R. DOE	123456	1-27-90	12-29-89	1-20-90 ⑮	1

IF YOU HAVE ANY QUESTIONS ABOUT THIS STATEMENT CALL:

BETTY BILLER PHONE 464-1234 MONDAY THROUGH FRIDAY 8:30 - 4:30

SERVICE DATE		DESCRIPTION	TOTAL AMOUNT	INSURANCE PORTION	PATIENT PORTION
		SUMMARY OF CHARGES ⑦			
12-29-89	120	ROOM & DAILY CARE			
		23 DAYS @$320/day 12-29-89 to 1-20-90	7360.00		
12-29-89	115	PATIENT TRAY-TOWELS, PILLOW, SLIPPERS	370.00		
1-2-90	250	PHARMACY	427.00		
1-4-90	258	IV SOLUTIONS ⑧	1052.00		
1-4-90	260	IV THERAPY	632.50		
1-4-90	270	MEDICAL-SURGICAL SUPPLIES	9.50		
1-2-90	300	LABORATORY	214.50		
1-5-90	301	LABORATORY/CHEMISTRY	63.00		
1-9-90	302	LABORATORY/IMMUNOLOGY	583.00		
1-11-90	305	LABORATORY/HEMATOLOGY	189.00		
1-15-90	306	LABORATORY/BACTERIOLOGY-MICROBIOLOGY	308.00		
1-17-90	307	LABORATORY/UROLOGY	154.50		
12-27-89	309	LABORATORY/PREADMISSION TESTING ⑨	480.00		
1-2-90	320	DIAGNOSTIC X-RAY	27.00		
1-2-90	320	DIAGNOSTIC X-RAY	27.00		
1-3-90	324	DIAGNOSTIC X-RAY/CHEST	213.50		
1-4-90	360	OPERATING ROOM SERVICES ⑩	90.00		
1-4-90	370	ANESTHESIA	452.00		
12-30-89	390	BLOOD/STORAGE PROCEDURES	20.00		
1-5-90	410	RESPIRATORY SERVICES	376.50		
1-8-90	420	PHYSICAL THERAPY	73.00		
1-4-90	710	RECOVERY ROOM	59.00		
1-3-90	730	ELECTROCARDIOGRAM	147.00		
1-20-90	999	ADMISSION/DISCHARGE PROCESSING	160.00		
⑪		TOTAL CHARGES ⑫	$13488.00		
		AMOUNT BILLED TO INSURANCE		$9961.20	⑭
⑬		PAY THIS AMOUNT			$3526.80

THANK YOU FOR CHOOSING JEFFERSON HEALTH SERVICES FOR YOUR MEDICAL CARE.

FINAL DIAGNOSIS	PLEASE READ REVERSE SIDE OF THIS STATEMENT
ACUTE ENDOCARDITIS	

Figure 4

(This line may contain the name of the patient or the patient's spouse. Hospitals want this information even though an insurance company may be paying the bill. They claim that their agreement to provide services is with the patient and not an insurance company.)

7. Does the hospital bill contain a description of services and a summary of charges for each department?

8. Do any of the individual department charges appear to be higher than they ought to be? (If the hospital billing clerk hits the wrong key, that $37 patient tray kit could end up costing $370.)

9. Do any preadmission testing charges appear on the bill? (Preadmission testing is billed separately and should not be listed on your hospital bill.)

10. Do any of the items listed in the "summary of charges" column appear more than once? (If you only had one chest X ray during your stay, you don't want to be billed for three chest X rays.)

11. Are the dates of services clearly indicated on the billing statement? (You'll need to have this information if there's a dispute over the bill with either the hospital or your insurance company.)

12. Does the billing statement contain a charge for admission or discharge processing? (Ideally, you should check with your doctor before you're admitted to determine what you will be receiving for these extra charges. The question here is really whether you get *anything* for your money. Very often these charges are little more than the hospital's paper processing fees. You can, however, request that these charges be taken off, but it is best to negotiate all this ahead of time rather than haggle afterward.)

13. Does the amount shown in the "estimated insurance payment" column match the payment schedule as shown on your insurance policy's schedule of benefits? (Many hospitals can tell you how much your insurance company will pay for the care you receive.

The estimate is based on the contract the hospital has with your insurance company and your particular plan's coverage.)

14. Is the "patient amount due" column clearly labeled? (Some statements have multiple columns showing various balances due and insurance payments expected, and unless the patient portion of the bill is clearly labeled you might accidentally pay for something that is covered by insurance.)

15. Does the hospital bill contain instructions on how to obtain an itemized bill, inquire about specific charges, or request an audit?

CAN YOU READ YOUR MEDICAL CHART?

One thing medical people just love to do is abbreviate, especially on your chart and medical record. You see, they think no one else, except another doctor or nurse, will ever have occasion to look at what is written there, and they all know the code.

But what about you? Do you know the code? If not, your chart and records will be nothing but meaningless scribbles to you, and you'll be shut out from what your doctor is thinking about you, about your condition, and about your prognosis. And that's one more obstacle blocking your participation in your own medical care.

Check your ability to decipher medical abbreviations with this quiz. It's simple: Match the abbreviation in Column A with its definition in Column B. Then check the answer key to see how you've done.

COLUMN A		COLUMN B	
1.	a.	(a)	blood pressure
2.	Aq.	(b)	oxygen
3.	Bl. time	(c)	temperature, pulse, and respiration
4.	BM	(d)	with (*cum*)
5.	BP	(e)	nausea and vomiting
6.	Bx	(f)	chief complaint

COLUMN A	COLUMN B	
7. c̄	(g)	postoperative
8. CBC	(h)	intramuscular
9. CC	(i)	patient
10. cc	(j)	treatment
11. CXR	(k)	while pain lasts (*durum dolorem*)
12. d	(l)	negative
13. dur dolor	(m)	diagnosis
14. Dx	(n)	general anesthesia
15. febris	(o)	complete blood count
16. FH	(p)	give
17. Fx	(q)	bowel movement
18. GA	(r)	at bedtime (*hora somni*)
19. gravida	(s)	every
20. h	(t)	intake and output of fluids
21. h.s.	(u)	water
22. Hx	(v)	white blood cell count
23. I&D	(w)	murmur
24. IM	(x)	fever
25. I&O	(y)	before
26. IV	(z)	chest X ray
27. ⓜ	(aa)	none
28. neg.	(bb)	standard operating procedure
29. NPO	(cc)	after (*post*)
30. N&V	(dd)	present illness
31. O₂	(ee)	pregnant
32. o	(ff)	cubic centimeter
33. OOB	(gg)	family history
34. P; p̄	(hh)	red blood cell count
35. PI	(ii)	bleeding time
36. postop	(jj)	prescription; therapy
37. PR	(kk)	without (*sine*)
38. pt	(ll)	fracture
39. Px	(mm)	right away, immediately (*statim*)
40. q	(nn)	symptoms
41. RBC	(oo)	intravenous

COLUMN A	COLUMN B	
42. Rx	(pp)	*non per os* (nothing by mouth)
43. s̄	(qq)	pulse rate
44. SOP	(rr)	vital signs
45. stat	(ss)	biopsy
46. Sx	(tt)	history
47. TPR	(uu)	hour, hourly
48. Tx	(vv)	incision and drainage
49. VS	(ww)	prognosis
50. WBC	(xx)	out of bed

■ ANSWERS

1. —y	2. —u	3. —ii	4. —q	5. —a
6. —ss	7. —d	8. —o	9. —f	10. —ff
11. —z	12. —p	13. —k	14. —m	15. —x
16. —gg	17. —ll	18. —n	19. —ee	20. —uu
21. —r	22. —tt	23. —vv	24. —h	25. —t
26. —oo	27. —w	28. —l	29. —pp	30. —e
31. —b	32. —aa	33. —xx	34. —cc	35. —dd
36. —g	37. —qq	38. —i	39. —ww	40. —s
41. —hh	42. —jj	43. —kk	44. —bb	45. —mm
46. —nn	47. —c	48. —j	49. —rr	50. —v

■ SCORING

50–40: Bravo. You've got a strong handle on medicine's cryptic codes. Be sure to use that skill.

39–25: Good start. You have the foundation for a fine understanding of med-speak. A little brushing up on medical abbreviations is all you need to build a stronger medical vocabulary.

Below 25: Start studying. If you can't decipher the abbreviations on your medical chart and records, you're missing a fundamental opportunity for participating in your medical care.

CAN YOU READ YOUR PRESCRIPTION FORM?

How often have you been given prescription forms, those little slips of paper with a jumble of foreign symbols and strangely abbreviated terms? And how often have you been able to read what the prescription says? Contrary to the message the medical establishment tries to convey, you don't need an M.D., R.N., or Pharm.D. degree to understand a prescription form. All you need is prescription-abbreviation savvy.

That's what this test is about. Match each medical abbreviation in Column A with the appropriate definition in Column B. Then check the scoring to see how well you translate prescription shorthand codes.

COLUMN A	COLUMN B
1. ac	(a) prescription; therapy
2. ad lib	(b) as often as necessary (*pro re nata*)
3. agit	(c) continue the medicine (*continuate remedium*)
4. bid	(d) of each (*singularis*)
5. c̄	(e) at bedtime (*hora somni*)
6. cap(s)	(f) once a day
7. cont rem	(g) as needed, as desired (*ad libitum*)
8. Disp.	(h) ointment (*unguentum*)
9. dur dolor	(i) daily
10. emp	(j) every morning
11. ext	(k) milligrams
12. gm	(l) orally (by mouth) (*per os*)
13. gtt	(m) capsule(s)
14. h	(n) while pain lasts (*durum dolorem*)
15. h.s.	(o) as directed
16. i	(p) four times a day
17. ii	(q) tablet(s)
18. iii	(r) one
19. ind	(s) every two hours
20. m et n	(t) grams

COLUMN A	COLUMN B
21. mg	(u) three times a day (*ter in die*)
22. ml	(v) under the tongue (*sub lingua*)
23. mor dict	(w) three
24. non rep; nr	(x) milliliter
25. O.D.	(y) with (*cum*)
26. pc	(z) do not repeat (*non repetite*)
27. pil	(aa) before meals (*ante cenum*)
28. po	(bb) dispense
29. pr	(cc) after meals (*post cenum*)
30. prn	(dd) apply topically
31. qam	(ee) times
32. qd	(ff) shake, stir (*agitate*)
33. qh	(gg) as directed (*ut dictum*)
34. q2h	(hh) by rectum (*per rectum*)
35. qhs	(ii) daily (*in dies*)
36. qid	(jj) every hour
37. qn	(kk) two
38. qod	(ll) every night
39. Rx	(mm) morning and night
40. sig	(nn) write, let it be imprinted (*signate*)
41. sing	(oo) twice a day (*bis die*)
42. sl	(pp) dissolve (*solvete*)
43. solv	(qq) hour, hourly
44. tab(s)	(rr) drops (*guttae*)
45. tid	(ss) in the manner directed (*more dicto*)
46. tinc.; tinct.	(tt) for external use
47. top	(uu) at hour of sleep
48. ung; ungt	(vv) tincture
49. ut dict	(ww) every other day
50. x	(xx) pill

■ **ANSWERS**

1. —aa	2. —g	3. —ff	4. —oo	5. —y
6. —m	7. —c	8. —bb	9. —n	10. —gg or c
11. —tt	12. —t	13. —rr	14. —qq	15. —e
16. —r	17. —kk	18. —w	19. —ii	20. —mm
21. —k	22. —x	23. —ss	24. —z	25. —f
26. —cc	27. —xx	28. —l	29. —hh	30. —b
31. —j	32. —i	33. —jj	34. —s	35. —uu
36. —p	37. —ll	38. —ww	39. —a	40. —nn
41. —d	42. —v	43. —pp	44. —q	45. —u
46. —vv	47. —dd	48. —h	49. —gg or o	50. —ee

■ **SCORING**

50–40: Excellent. No medical abbreviation will intimidate you, for you have the key to understanding medical codes.

39–25: Good start. You know the basics of prescription abbreviations, but there's room for improvement.

Below 25: Prescription abbreviations are still a deep, dark secret. It's time to learn some of medicine's most common abbreviations and codes. Don't leave yourself in the dark.

INSURANCE QUIZ

Do you understand the lingo of the insurance industry? If not, join the legions of people equally confused and befuddled. However, as more and more businesses change their medical benefits plans, you may find it necessary to learn the language of insurance in self-defense. The insurance field is a jungle of sound-alike terms. The better you know what they really mean, the less likely you are to buy a policy you don't want or need and waste that precious commodity, money, only to end up underinsured.

Examine the terms in Part A and then select the terms from Part B that best define them. Some of these terms have similar-sounding definitions—why should we make it easy when the insurance industry doesn't?—so make sure you read them carefully.

■ PART A

1. Preexisting condition
2. Exclusions
3. Conversion clause
4. Deductible
5. Grace period
6. Schedule of benefits

7. Third-party payer
8. Free-look period
9. Copayment
10. Stop-loss
11. Premium
12. Rider
13. Indemnity policy
14. Service contract
15. Major medical insurance

16. Actuary
17. Cancellation
18. Coordination of benefits
19. Waiting period
20. Benefits
21. Usual, customary, and reasonable
22. Limitations
23. Assignment
24. Contributory
25. Risk
26. Effective date
27. Prepaid plan
28. Inside limit
29. Policy limit
30. Lapsed policy

■ PART B

(a) A person professionally trained to apply probability and statistics to problems of the insurance industry.

(b) The signed transfer of policy benefits to a party other than the insured—for example, a doctor or hospital.

(c) The amount payable in either cash or services to you or some beneficiary under the provisions of an insurance policy.

(d) The termination of an existing policy before it would normally expire.

(e) A provision found in health insurance policies that requires you and the insurance company to share the cost of a covered service.

(f) A provision of group insurance plans that requires both employer and employee to contribute to the cost of the plan.

(g) The privilege granted by a group policy to convert to an individual policy upon termination of group coverage.

(h) A practice used by insurance companies to determine their liability for a claim when you are covered by more than one policy.

(i) An out-of-pocket payment that must be met before your policy begins to pay benefits.

(j) The date on which a claim may be filed and benefits will be paid.

(k) Specific conditions or services that are not covered and for which no benefits will be paid—for example, routine office visits.

(l) A period of time, usually 10 to 30 days, during which you may cancel a newly purchased insurance policy and have your money fully refunded.

(m) A period of time, usually 30 or 31 days, after the date a premium is due, during which the insurance policy remains in force and the premium may still be paid.

(n) A health insurance policy that pays a specific amount of money for hospital and physician services. Generally, this amount does not cover the entire cost of the care provided.

(o) A provision found in some insurance policies that limits the amount of payment that is made for a service regardless of the total cost of that service—for example, a $500 limit on all surgical procedures.

(p) An insurance policy that has been terminated and is no longer in force.

(q) A clause that limits coverage under certain circumstances (such as war) or certain illnesses.

(r) A health insurance policy designed to offset the large expenses of catastrophic illness or injury.

(s) The maximum benefits a particular policy will pay.

(t) A physical and/or mental condition which you have and/or had before you applied for insurance.

(u) The payment required to keep a policy in force.

(v) A plan that pays hospitals and doctors for medical services before they are needed or delivered.

(w) A document that amends a policy or certificate.

(x) Any chance of a loss.

(y) A list that details what services a particular insurance policy covers, such as dollar limits, exclusions, and policy limits.

(z) An insurance plan that has a contract with hospitals and/or doctors and pays them according to an agreed-upon fee schedule for medical services provided.

(aa) A provision of an insurance policy that limits your out-of-pocket expenses to a set amount, after which the insurance company pays all costs.

(bb) Any public or private organization, such as an insurance company, that reimburses hospitals and doctors for services provided to policyholders.

(cc) A term applied to charges for medical care that are consistent with the going rate or charges in a certain geographical area for identical or similar services.

(dd) The length of time an employee must wait, from his or her date of employment or application, before his or her policy will pay a claim.

■ **ANSWERS**

1. —t	2. —k	3. —g	4. —i	5. —m
6. —y	7. —bb	8. —l	9. —e	10. —aa
11. —u	12. —w	13. —n	14. —z	15 —r
16. —a	17. —d	18. —h	19. —dd	20. —c
21. —cc	22. —q	23. —b	24. —f	25. —x
26. —j	27. —v	28. —o	29. —s	30. —p

MEDICARE: WHAT DO YOU KNOW?

Medicare is the largest and, without a doubt, the most complicated insurance program ever designed. And with good reason—it was put together by a committee.

As any Medicare beneficiary can tell you, Medicare coverage is a maze of innumerable rules and regulations, inexplicable exceptions and limitations, and constantly changing forms and filing procedures. Yet it's hardly a cheap proposition—for anyone concerned. The federal government is spending in excess of $100 billion a year to fund Medicare, and beneficiaries—that's you, if you are 65 or older—are spending another $3 billion. Then there's the multibillion-dollar supplemental insurance industry that costs beneficiaries anywhere from $60 to $100 a month for supplemental insurance (for what's *not* covered by the feds).

Let's test how much you know about the system. Whether you're a Medicare beneficiary yourself or are just following along because you'll soon be there, knowing merely the basics is a good start at ensuring that you (or someone in your family) will get the most out of the Medicare program—in short, will get what you're entitled to. To give you an even chance, we've made it a true-or-false quiz. True or false:

1. To be eligible for Medicare, a person must be at least 65 years of age or older.

2. To be eligible for Medicare, a person must be entitled to payment under the Social Security Act or Railroad Retirement Act.

3. A nonworking spouse is eligible for Medicare even though the working spouse died before reaching age 65.

4. Medicare may be purchased by those unable to qualify for coverage under present law.

5. An application for Medicare may not be made until a person's 65th birthday.

6. When a person applies for Medicare and is deemed eligible, he or she is automatically enrolled in Medicare Part B (medical insurance).

7. Medicare Part A is very often referred to as hospital insurance.

8. Medicare is administered by the Social Security Administration.

9. Medicare Part B is provided free of charge to those people eligible for Medicare Part A.

10. Medicare Part A requires the payment of an annual deductible.

11. The deductible for Medicare Part A has increased every year since coverage began.

12. The deductible for Medicare Part B must be met before coverage begins.

13. Medicare assignment is when the hospital, doctor, or laboratory accepts the Medicare-approved amount as payment in full.

14. The majority of doctors in this country accept Medicare assignment on all of their claims.

15. When a doctor accepts Medicare assignment, he or she receives 80 percent of the payment from Medicare and 20 percent from the Medicare beneficiary.

16. Medicare Part A covers all types of nursing-home care.

17. Medicare reimburses hospitals on the basis of what is known as a Diagnosis Related Group (DRG) system.

18. When a Medicare patient enters the hospital, he or she must be advised of his or her discharge rights.

19. Hospitals may discharge Medicare patients once the government's predetermined payment levels have been reached.

20. If notified that the hospital intends to discharge them, Medicare hospital patients may apply to the peer review organization.

21. Medicare provides an unlimited number of days of hospital care.

22. Medicare pays the total cost of skilled nursing-facility care for the first twenty days.

23. Medicare coverage of prescription drugs was deleted when catastrophic coverage was repealed in 1990.

24. Medicare does not provide for any medical coverage in foreign countries.

25. An Explanation of Medicare Benefits (EOMB) is sent to a beneficiary whenever a service is provided under Medicare Part B.

26. Medigap, or supplemental, insurance duplicates and expands Medicare coverage.

27. Medicare provides an unlimited number of days of hospice care (care for the terminally ill).

28. Medicare beneficiaries are eligible to join a health maintenance organization if there is one near where they live.

29. Balance billing—charging more than the Medicare-approved amount—is the practice used by physicians who do not accept Medicare assignment.

30. Medicare now provides coverage for over-the-counter drugs, hearing aids, and routine eye exams.

31. Medicare beneficiaries should carry more than one supplemental policy to ensure maximum protection.

32. Medicare beneficiaries can find the names of doctors in their areas who accept assignment by contacting their nearest Social Security Administration office.

33. The Peer Review Organization (PRO) is responsible for determining whether or not a Medicare beneficiary may be admitted to a hospital for an outpatient procedure.

34. A Medicare beneficiary cannot be retroactively charged for medical services that are later deemed to be inappropriate.

35. If your request for payment under Medicare Part B is denied, your only recourse is to pay for the service out of your own pocket.

36. If a person becomes eligible for Medicare *and* continues to work, he or she may be dropped from his or her employer's medical insurance plan.

37. A person who is diagnosed as having end-stage renal (kidney) disease is eligible for Medicare.

38. Medicare covers skilled-nursing facility care after a person has been hospitalized for at least three days.

39. The Medicare program provides a maximum of sixty lifetime reserve hospital days per beneficiary.

40. Private-duty nursing is covered under Medicare Part A.

■ **ANSWERS**

1. False.

   Medicare is also available to those who are permanently and totally disabled and those who have end-stage renal disease.

2. True.

   But beyond being entitled to payment under the Social Security Act or the Railroad Retirement Act, you must meet a citizenship requirement.

3. True.

   According to the law, widows and widowers are both eligible if they are over 65 years of age.

4. True.

   Medicare Parts A and B may be purchased if you are otherwise ineligible for coverage, but you must first meet age requirements. Check with an office of the Social Security Administration for information on the current premium.

5. False.

   You may apply for your Medicare benefits three months before or after your 65th birthday.

6. False.

   You are not automatically enrolled in Medicare Part B when you apply for Part A. If you miss the general enrollment period during your first period of eligibility, you will end up paying a financial penalty in the form of higher Part B premiums.

7. True.

   Medicare Part A is known as hospital insurance, because it covers hospital services. Medicare Part B, which is the medical insurance portion, covers physician and other outpatient services.

8. False.

   The Health Care Financing Administration operates the Medicare program, while the Social Security Administration is responsible for eligibility requirements.

9. False.

Medicare beneficiaries must pay a monthly premium for Medicare Part B. This premium is automatically deducted from your Social Security check.

10. False.

The deductible for Medicare Part A is on a per incident basis, which means that every time you are admitted to the hospital, you must pay the one-day deductible. However, should you be readmitted to the hospital within sixty days of your first admission, you would not be responsible for the deductible.

11. True.

The Medicare Part A deductible has increased every year since 1966 and now stands at over $600 per incident.

12. True.

Medicare Part B begins to cover physician expenses after you have met the $100 deductible.

13. True.

Medicare assignment means that the provider (physician, lab, or whatever) accepts the Medicare-approved amount as payment in full. Medicare pays 80 percent and you pay 20 percent.

14. False.

According to statistics compiled by the Health Care Financing Administration, fewer than 45 percent of doctors accept Medicare assignment on all of their claims.

15. True.

Medicare reimburses the doctor at 80 percent of the approved amount, and you are responsible for the remaining 20 percent of the payment.

16. False.

Medicare Part A does not cover intermediate or custodial care but instead provides limited coverage for a skilled-nursing facility.

17. True.

The Diagnosis Related Group (DRG) system is the basic method Medicare uses to pay hospitals for services provided to Medicare beneficiaries. All diagnoses are assigned a certain dollar value and a length of stay. The hospital receives the assigned amount regardless of the actual cost of your care or length of stay.

18. True.

As a result of action taken by the People's Medical Society and the American Association of Retired Persons, all Medicare patients must be advised in writing of their discharge rights upon admission to the hospital.

19. False.

A hospital cannot discharge you just because your stay may be longer or more costly than the reimbursement the hospital will receive from Medicare under the DRG system.

20. True.

You should contact the Peer Review Organization immediately upon being notified that the hospital intends to discharge you. The PRO has the authority to review your case and determine whether or not there is a medically justified reason for discharging you. The hospital will tell you how to contact the PRO.

21. False.

Medicare provides a maximum of ninety hospital days per benefit period and a maximum of sixty lifetime reserve days. Once you use a lifetime reserve day, it is never replaced.

22. True.

Following a three-day hospital stay, Medicare will cover the first twenty days of skilled nursing facility care. Your copayment begins on the twenty-first day.

23. True.

The prescription drug coverage scheduled to go into effect was canceled with the repeal of the catastrophic-coverage bill. No prescription drugs are reimbursable under Medicare.

24. True.

Medicare covers only hospital care delivered in the United States. Under emergency conditions, it will cover care in Canadian and Mexican hospitals, but only if they are the closest facilities available.

25. True.

You will receive your Explanation of Medicare Benefits (EOMB) from the Medicare carrier for your state. It will indicate the name of the provider, the type of care, the Medicare-approved amount, the Medicare payment, and the amount you owe.

26. False.

A Medicare supplemental policy should not duplicate Medicare coverage. It is designed to fill in the gaps in the Medicare program and may offer additional services.

27. False.

Hospice care is limited to a total of 210 days with two ninety-day periods and one thirty-day period of care.

28. True.

To be eligible for a Medicare HMO, you must be enrolled in Medicare Parts A and B, live in the service area of the HMO, and enroll during the open enrollment period. You cannot be an end-stage renal disease patient and must not be receiving hospice care.

29. True.

Medicare beneficiaries pay some $3 billion a year in excess charges because the majority of doctors do not accept Medicare assignment. As a result of balance billing, Medicare beneficiaries spend an average of nearly 18 percent of their income for medical services.

30. False.

Medicare does not cover over-the-counter drugs, hearing aids, or routine eye exams.

31. False.

Additional supplemental policies do nothing but cost you money. One comprehensive supplemental policy is all that you need.

32. True.

Your local office of the Social Security Administration maintains a directory with the names of doctors who accept assignment.

33. True.

The Peer Review Organization will determine whether or not your admission to the hospital for an outpatient procedure can be medically justified.

34. True.

If your Medicare carrier (the insurance company in your state that processes the Medicare Part B claims) or the Peer Review Organization determines that a service you received was inappropriate, it may deny payment to the doctor. Since you could not be expected to know if a service was appropriate or inappropriate, the doctor may not retroactively collect the fee from you.

35. False.

You have the right to appeal a denial of your claim. Contact your Medicare carrier and obtain a copy of HCFA form 1964, Request for Review of Part B Medicare Claims.

36. False.

Medicare regulations mandate that your employer continue to carry you on the company medical benefits plan. In this case Medicare becomes your secondary carrier and will supplement your employer's medical plan.

37. True.

Due to the excessive cost of dialysis, Congress determined that a person diagnosed as having end-stage renal disease is eligible for Medicare coverage.

38. True.

    The requirement is a three-day hospital stay.

39. True.

    Medicare currently provides a maximum of sixty lifetime reserve hospital days. Once used, these days are not replenished.

40. False.

    Medicare does not provide for private-duty nursing.

■ SCORING

40–36: Excellent. You understand the workings of the Medicare system and know how to avoid problems and make it work. You might consider sharing your knowledge with less informed Medicare beneficiaries.

35–31: Very good. Medicare may present a lot of problems for others, but you've shown that you know a thing or two about the system. You could easily move up to the top score with a little review of Medicare material.

30–21: Good. You know the answers to more than half of the questions. Another review of the federal government's booklet *Your Medicare Handbook* and the People's Medical Society's *Medicare Made Easy*, and you'll challenge the top scores.

DO YOU KNOW YOUR MEDICAL RECORD RIGHTS?

From its very inception, the People's Medical Society has demanded that consumers have access to their medical records. After all, we can't be smart consumers if we can't see the most basic data about our own health. Unfortunately, many doctors and hospitals are reluctant to share medical records, claiming that you might not understand their notes or that you might be frightened away from a "needed" procedure.

Let's find out how much you know about your medical record—so that you know how to go to bat for your rights.

1. A medical record is
   (a) a folder in a doctor's office that includes data about your health, a description of your medical history, notes from physical exams, X rays and charts, and results of tests that you've had.
   (b) a sheaf of papers in a hospital that includes reports from hospital departments that have treated you, doctors' notes on your health, medical history, and physical exams, X rays and charts, and consent forms.
   (c) sheets of paper or forms that you keep at home and on which you record information about your medical history, visits to doctors' offices, hospitalizations, laboratory tests, dental and eye examinations, and prescription and nonprescription medications you are taking.
   (d) all of the above.
2. Medical records serve as guideposts for determining the course of your medical care.
   (a) True
   (b) False
3. It's important to have access to your medical records because
   (a) doctors write things in there that they don't always tell you.
   (b) many medical records have errors, and if you see the records, you may be able to correct the inaccuracies.
   (c) both of the above are true.
4. Errors in medical records are caused by
   (a) physicians omitting important information.
   (b) laboratory and hospital personnel errors.
   (c) misinformation from patients.
   (d) all of the above.
5. In most states, you are entitled to
   (a) the original medical record, including charts and X rays.
   (b) copies of the medical record, including charts and X rays.
   (c) both of the above.
6. Consumers have a *legal* right to full access to physician, hospital, and mental health records
   (a) sometimes.

(b) always.

(c) never.

■ **ANSWERS**

1. (d) All three of these are forms of medical records. And all three of them are valuable sources of information about your health. Hospital records and charts (usually kept at the nurses' station) are somewhat difficult to get hold of, and you have to make a special request to your doctor to see his or her record. But you can easily keep an accurate record of your medical history, and that record will always be at hand.

2. (a) True. Medical records are accorded great authority by the medical system. In some cases, doctors spend more time with your medical records than they spend with you.

3. (c) There are plenty of reasons to examine your medical record occasionally, not the least of which is to find out what's really going on. Your record can be an especially important minivolume of facts and figures if your doctor or the hospital staff isn't being clear in explaining your condition, or seems reticent in giving you information about yourself. And, yes, errors occur in records—and who's to correct the mistake if you're not there to point it out?

4. (d) Medical records have long been marred by errors, according to John F. Burnum, M.D., writing in "The Misinformation Age: The Fall of the Medical Record" (*Annals of Internal Medicine*, March 15, 1989). Says Burnum: "At the very time information machines are becoming more important, the information transferred is getting worse. All medical record information should be regarded as suspect; much of it is fiction."

5. (b) In most states, you are entitled to copies of your medical record (usually if you are willing to pay reasonable copying costs). The originals are the property of the doctor or hospital. This doesn't mean that a doctor can't share an X ray, for example, with another physician. It's just that the first doctor retains ownership of the original material.

6. (a) We say "sometimes" because your medical record rights vary

from state to state. Some states grant consumers full access to all medical records; others will grant access only under certain conditions; still other states have no provision for consumer access at all. But even if access laws are not on the books in your state, your doctor can certainly—and legally—share your records with you. A good doctor should be eager to keep you informed.

DO YOU KNOW YOUR PENSION RIGHTS?

It's only human nature that the closer you get to retirement age, the more important your pension benefits become to you. Many people consider retirement as that time of their lives when they can sit back and relax, secure in the knowledge that their pension check will arrive right on schedule. However, unless you know your pension rights, what should be a time of peace and security can be fraught with worry and apprehension. With mergers, takeovers, and buy-outs more and more a part of the business climate, today's pensioners-to-be face a rocky road to retirement security. And that's only part of the pension security concern.

Do you know the necessary steps to ensure that your spouse will receive survivor benefits should something happen to you? If you are a woman, are you at higher risk of losing pension benefits than men are? Does the federal government provide any type of pension benefit guarantee? Does your pension plan meet or exceed the minimum requirements of qualified pension plans? Do you fully understand the vesting requirements of your pension? Do you know the difference between a defined benefit plan and a defined contribution plan?

Today some 50 million workers are covered by various forms of private pension plans, and each worker is counting on having that pension benefit available upon retirement. To help ensure that the big day arrives, Congress has passed various laws on pension plan rights and protections. This is especially critical for women, who all too often lose pension benefits because they haven't been in pension plans long enough to be fully vested or because their monthly payment is based on an earnings record that hasn't been adjusted for inflation or cost-of-living changes. Knowing how to evaluate your pension plan will not only improve your financial health; it will also prevent you from worrying yourself sick.

Your employer is required to furnish you with specific information on the legal organization of your pension fund and the name of the plan administrator. If you have not been supplied with this type of information, it could jeopardize your pension benefits and rights. Take the following quiz to learn how well you know and understand the regulations governing pension plans. True or false:

1. The Employee Retirement Income Security Act of 1974—popularly referred to as ERISA—requires your employer to provide you with a qualified pension plan.

2. State and federal workers are covered by federal pension plan laws.

3. Employers who offer pension plans are permitted by federal law to exclude employees who work less than twenty hours a week or 1,000 hours a year.

4. A qualified pension plan is one that meets the minimum standards for pension coverage, funding, reporting, and disclosure as defined by the Employee Retirement Income Security Act of 1974.

5. In the event your company goes out of business or is bought by another firm, you stand to lose all of your pension benefits.

6. As a participant in a qualified pension plan, your plan administrator is required by federal law to provide you with copies of documents with specific information on an annual basis.

7. Your plan administrator will automatically send you information on your benefits at least once a year.

8. When you are "vested" in your retirement plan, it means that you have earned a legal right to your pension benefits.

9. Qualified pension plans are required to provide you with information on vesting, and the time it requires for you to become fully vested in the plan.

10. If you are within a few years of normal retirement age (65), your employer has the right to exclude you from participating in the company pension plan.

11. Employees who reach their pension plan's normal retirement age automatically become fully vested, even if they have less than the required years of service in the plan.

12. A defined contribution plan is designed to pay you a specified dollar amount when you retire, such as $100 a month.

13. Monthly pension benefits are usually determined by a formula that can be found in the plan's Summary Annual Report.

14. The most commonly used method for computing monthly pension benefits is a combination of the following factors: your age at retirement, your type of plan, your earnings in a salary-related plan, and your years of service.

15. Your pension benefits may be reduced by up to one-half when you are also receiving Social Security benefits.

16. The Retirement Equity Act of 1984 guarantees a woman the right to collect her pension benefits or her husband's benefits in the event he dies before or after retirement.

17. Pension plans that provide retirement benefits in the form of annuities must provide survivor benefits.

18. A spouse is entitled to survivor benefits if the working spouse made the request in writing at the time of application for retirement benefits.

19. Survivor benefits must be paid to the spouse of a deceased plan participant even if he or she was not fully vested at the time of death.

20. Survivor benefits must be paid to the spouse of a fully vested plan participant who dies before retirement age.

21. When a fully vested plan participant dies after retirement, the survivor annuity payment must be at least 50 percent of the regular monthly benefit and must continue until the survivor dies.

22. Federal law requires that pension-plan funds be treated as an asset of the marriage and be divided in the event of a divorce.

23. A woman who enters and leaves the work force during her working years, even though she worked the same number of years as a man, typically receives a lower monthly benefit.

24. Many married couples waive surviving-spouse benefits in order to receive larger monthly benefits while they are both living.

25. If your company decides to terminate your pension plan, it may do so without notifying you.

■ **ANSWERS**

1. False.

There are no federal or state laws that require your employer to provide you with a pension plan. An employer's decision to provide pension benefits is purely voluntary.

2. False.

Federal and state workers are not covered by federal pension laws. The law only applies to private employers.

3. True.

Federal law does permit part-time workers to be excluded from participating in pension plans. This mostly affects women, who comprise about 66 percent of the part-time work force.

4. True.

The Employee Retirement Income Security Act of 1974 sets the standards for the operation of qualified pension plans.

5. False.

Your pension benefits are protected by the Pension Benefit Guaranty Corporation, the U.S. Department of Labor, and the Internal Revenue Service.

6. True.

You must receive the Summary Plan Description, Summary Annual Report, and Survivor Coverage Data from your plan administrator at least once a year.

7. Not necessarily true.

In many cases, you must submit a written request in order to obtain a copy of your Individual Benefit Statement, available once a year.

8. True.

"To vest" means to put someone into authority or control over something ("a vested interest"); in insurance usage, it indicates that the beneficiary has earned the right to collect the benefits of his or her retirement plan after a certain number of years of participating in the plan.

9. True.

There are two types of vesting used by pension plans. *Cliff vesting* (an all-or-nothing vesting method) in single-employer plans must occur after five years of service. The beneficiary does not earn any portion of pension benefits until the fifth year of service, at which time full vesting occurs. If the person leaves a job anytime before the fifth year of service, he or she loses all benefits. In multi-employer plans (plans formed by a specific industry, such as logging, or a group of smaller companies), full vesting must occur no later than after ten years of service.

Graded vesting (earning a percentage of pension benefits during a set period of time) requires that participants must earn at least 20 percent vested rights after three years of service. An additional 20 percent vesting must be earned during each of the next four years. Full vesting must occur no later than the end of the seventh year.

10. False.

You may not be excluded from participating in a pension plan because you are too old or because you were hired within a few years of the plan's normal retirement age.

11. True.

Employees who reach their pension plan's normal retirement age automatically become fully vested, even if they have less than the required number of years of service.

12. False.

A defined *benefit* plan and not a defined *contribution* plan promises to pay a specified monthly benefit at retirement—for example, $200.

13. False.

The Summary Plan Description and not the Summary Annual Report contains the formula for computing the monthly pension benefit.

14. True.

Pension plans typically use these factors to determine the monthly benefit.

15. True.

This is called integration of benefits, which means that your monthly pension payment may be reduced up to one-half if you are also receiving Social Security benefits. This has historically affected more women than men.

16. True.

The Retirement Equity Act of 1984 makes survivor benefits automatic and offers some new ways for women to protect themselves against losing their own or their husbands' pension benefits.

17. True.

By law, pension plans that offer benefits in the form of annuities (monthly payments) must provide for survivor benefits.

18. False.

The only way a woman would not receive her deceased husband's pension benefits is if she signed a written and notarized agreement waiving her survivor benefits.

19. True.

The law requires that survivor benefits be paid to the surviving spouse even though the deceased spouse was not fully vested. The only exception would be if both spouses waived the survivor benefit option.

20. True.

Survivor benefits must be paid to the spouse of a fully vested participant who dies before reaching retirement age. However, the annuity payments to the surviving spouse may not begin until the date the deceased spouse would have reached the plan's earliest retirement age. For example, if the participating spouse dies at age 50 and the plan's earliest retirement age is 55, the surviving spouse has to wait another five years to collect benefits.

21. True.

If a plan participant dies after retirement, his or her spouse must receive at least 50 percent of the annuity payment they had been receiving together.

22. False.

The Retirement Equity Act of 1984 authorizes courts to consider a pension plan as property of a marriage, but does not require them to do so. It also allows courts to award survivor benefits to parties involved in a divorce.

23. True.

Pension benefits are generally calculated on final earnings, when workers are expected to be at the top of their pay scale. This works fine for those people who stay in the same job and don't have any breaks in their service; however, women tend to leave the work force more often than men and, therefore, never achieve the higher earnings of the later years. This has the chilling effect of reducing their monthly pension benefit to one-half of a man's benefits.

24. True.

Many couples continue to waive the surviving spouse benefits because they want to receive higher monthly benefits while they are both alive. Generally, when survivor benefits are calculated, the monthly payment is lower, since the benefits are paid out over a longer period of time.

25. False.

Federal law requires that your plan administrator notify you at least sixty days in advance of the pension plan being terminated. This notice must be in writing and must tell you the amount of your benefit, as well as the method used to compute your benefit.

■ SCORING

25–21: Excellent. You've demonstrated that you know your ERISA and REA regulations like the back of your hand. You won't have any problems protecting your pension rights.

20–16: Good. Review the questions you missed to determine why you missed them and bone up on those particular aspects of pension rules and regulations.

15 or less: Poor. You need to get a copy of the Summary Plan Description and study the regulations and policies that apply to your plan. If you don't, you could be headed for real trouble when it comes time to file a retirement claim.

MALPRACTICE SUITS: DO YOU KNOW THE FACTS FROM THE FICTION?

In print and over the airwaves, organized medicine has been decrying the "present malpractice crisis," an issue medicine calls the most serious problem facing practicing physicians today. On the other hand, the People's Medical Society has long believed that one of the most serious problems facing medical consumers today is the issue of quality of care—the very fact of malpractice itself.

How much do you know about malpractice—and the ways it can affect your health care? Take this quiz and find out.

1. Malpractice lawsuits are
   (a) frivolous claims for unavoidable and unfortunate injuries, designed to force insurance companies to fork over large sums to consumers.

(b) meritorious claims for compensation for the harm caused by a practitioner's or institution's departure from accepted medical standards.

2. The *real* cause of malpractice suits is
   (a) greedy, vindictive consumers.
   (b) incompetent and irresponsible doctors.
   (c) litigation-happy lawyers.
   (d) all of the above.

3. The United States is in the midst of a malpractice crisis because the number of malpractice claims and the dollar awards to victims are skyrocketing.
   (a) true
   (b) false

4. Increases in huge jury settlements are driving insurance costs up.
   (a) true
   (b) false

5. Which of the following is NOT one of the five most frequently reported malpractice claims?
   (a) surgery/postoperative complications
   (b) improper treatment/birth-related
   (c) failure to diagnose cancer
   (d) surgery/inadvertent act
   (e) anesthesia/cardiac arrest

6. The percentage of patients' malpractice claims resulting in no awards or financial settlements is
   (a) 12.8 percent
   (b) 39.3 percent
   (c) 56.7 percent
   (d) 71.5 percent

7. Most malpractice takes place
   (a) in hospitals.
   (b) in doctors' offices.

8. Who is most frequently named in medical malpractice claims?
   (a) hospitals
   (b) doctors

9. To avoid lawsuits, physicians should
   (a) conduct as many tests as possible so that the diagnosis or course of action is unquestionable.
   (b) discuss treatment options with the patient and admit the error if anything goes wrong.
   (c) subscribe to a computerized service that indicates whether a patient has previously sued other doctors.
   (d) do all of the above.

10. Doctors who have had malpractice suits filed against them are not disciplined by physician licensing groups.
    (a) true
    (b) false

11. If you wish to stop a negligent doctor from harming anyone else, the best thing is
    (a) to complain to another doctor, particularly one who treats you.
    (b) to file a written complaint with your state's medical licensing board.
    (c) to complain in writing to your state senator or state representative.
    (d) to do all of the above.

■ ANSWERS

1. (b) Although insurance companies and some physicians like to paint a picture of malpractice suits as unreasonable and unwarranted actions, the fact is that many consumers are injured by unscrupulous, incompetent, or irresponsible doctors. And those consumers file suits because they want a truthful explanation and fair compensation for their injuries. And they want the doctor's incompetence exposed.

2. (b) Malpractice suits will continue as long as malpractitioners are allowed to practice their bad brand of medicine. Granted,

most doctors are competent and responsible and treat patients to the best of their ability. But a handful of incompetent and unscrupulous doctors continue to harm patients simply because the medical profession is unable or unwilling to police itself. Until the medical profession takes responsibility for this problem and regularly reprimands or expels malpractitioners, lawsuits will remain a fact of life.

3. (b) No matter how you slice it, the malpractice crisis seems to have peaked. According to data from Jury Verdict Research, Inc., the average malpractice award, the largest malpractice awards, and the number of million-dollar awards have all been declining. In fact, government investigation has found that some insurance companies *created* a malpractice crisis by unnecessarily raising doctors' premiums. For example, in one of the only comprehensive, multistate analyses of malpractice claims, the Minnesota Department of Commerce discovered that an insurer *tripled* doctors' malpractice premiums even though the number of claims against doctors *did not* go up.

4. (b) Juries are not the villains here. According to the Minnesota Department of Commerce investigation, fewer than one-half of 1 percent of all malpractice claimants were awarded damages by a jury. Most patients settle malpractice claims out of court.

5. (e) Based on 1987–88 data from St. Paul Fire and Marine Insurance, the largest private malpractice insurer in the country, there were only eighty-nine "allegations" of anesthesia/cardiac arrest, compared to 1,474 for postoperative complications from surgery, 661 for improper birth-related treatment, 607 for failure to diagnose cancer, and 375 for inadvertent acts of surgery.

6. (c) More than half of all malpractice claims—56.7 percent, to be exact—result in no award or financial settlement, according to a 1986 U.S. General Accounting Office (GAO) report, which gleaned its findings from a GAO review of 73,500 "closed" malpractice claims from twenty-five insurers.

7. (a) Statistics from St. Paul Fire and Marine Insurance for 1987–88 showed that 68 percent of the claims were the result of

injuries occurring in hospitals. The doctor's office was the setting for 28.7 percent of malpractice claims.

8. (b) Doctors are named in malpractice claims about 70 percent
of the time; hospitals are named in 21 percent, according to the
1986 General Accounting Office study.

9. (b) Doctors are learning that admitting an error, explaining
what happened, and apologizing can avoid a lawsuit. "Communi-
cating with the patient is probably the most important aspect
of loss prevention," a representative of the Physicians Insurance Association told a *Wall Street Journal* reporter (April 28,
1989).

10. (a) Sad to say this again, but the medical profession is unable
or unwilling to police itself. Even though a small percentage of
doctors is responsible for a high percentage of paid malpractice
claims, those doctors are rarely disciplined. A *Journal of the
American Medical Association* study of malpractice lawsuits in
Florida, for example, revealed that *none* of the doctors with
adverse claims experience had their licenses suspended or re-
voked in Florida, and that *more than 90 percent* of these physicians were never disciplined in any manner.

11. (d) All of the above. A surprisingly large number of consumers
file lawsuits and tell judge, jury, and lawyer that they don't
want any money; they just want to make sure that the guilty
physician is no longer allowed to practice. Although state licensing agencies or hospitals rarely revoke licenses or privileges,
you should put your complaint in writing to them, for the record. Also complain to your treating doctor if he or she wasn't
the cause of the problem. The doctor might be in the best
position to alert a medical board or a hospital administration to
the ticking time-bomb doctor. State (*not* federal) senators or
representatives can also pitch in and help your cause if you
make your case clear to them.

6. THE 21 MOST IMPORTANT HOME MEDICAL TESTS

Home medical testing has made it possible for people to take better care of themselves and thus remain healthier. The availability of sophisticated and reliable equipment has added a whole new emphasis to home medical tests. It's easy to forget that just a few short years ago, home testing was limited to taking body temperature.

Nowadays, computer-controlled devices are used to monitor heart rate and respiration, blood pressure, and blood sugar. Mechanical equipment can be used to measure the percentage of body fat, examine an eardrum for an infection, or illuminate a sinus cavity. Other chemical-based tests use specially treated paper, in the form of dipsticks, to test blood and urine.

Home medical testing is not designed to replace professional medical care; however, it can help you determine when you need professional care.

Not only are there more home-testing products on the market, but they are also more widely available. You'll find home tests at pharmacies, where they may be displayed in special sections, in health and beauty stores, and in supermarkets, and through mail-order companies. Home medical tests can give you the information you need to make informed decisions about your medical care and your overall health.

When used properly, home medical tests enable you to determine, monitor, and screen for various illnesses and conditions. However, there are precautions worth noting. Here are some consumer tips issued by the Food and Drug Administration. Keep these suggestions in mind when using all self-care test products.

1. Before you buy, note the expiration date for kits that contain chemicals. Don't buy a test if the expiration date is past.
2. Follow storage instructions. Keep containers tightly capped. Avoid moisture, light, and extremes of heat and cold. Keep out of reach of children.
3. Read and study the package insert. Make sure you understand the test and how to use it. Follow instructions exactly. Do not skip steps. If the test is timed, use a clock or a watch to be precise.
4. Note special precautions such as avoiding certain foods, drugs, or vitamins before testing. Take the test at the recommended time, if any is specified.
5. Some tests use colors to indicate results. If you are color-blind, have someone who can discern color help you interpret test results.
6. Some tests require collecting urine. Always collect urine in a clean, dry container. Soap or other residue can cause faulty test results.
7. Know what to do if test results are positive, negative, or unclear.
8. If you have questions about a test, consult a pharmacist or other health-care professional. Also, check the package insert for a telephone number you can call.

The following section describes what we consider to be the twenty-one most important home medical tests. Some of these tests require special equipment, while others do not. We'll describe the test, tell you how it's conducted, and suggest where it might be available.

BODY TEMPERATURE

Monitoring the body's temperature is probably the easiest home test there is, and one you've most likely done hundreds of times. The most common types of thermometers are the following.

ORAL GLASS BULB

The most popular type of thermometer, probably found in every home. Usually filled with mercury or some other heat-sensitive chemical. The mercury-filled thermometer appears to have a silver streak in the center, while the other chemical appears red.

ELECTRONIC THERMOMETER

A heat-sensitive metal tip is placed in the mouth and a mini-computer chip electronically reads and displays the temperature in digital form. This is usually the most expensive type of thermometer.

DISPOSABLE THERMOMETER

This thermometer is used once and discarded. It uses specially treated, heat-sensitive paper that either displays the actual temperature or changes color to indicate a fever is present.

PLASTIC STRIP THERMOMETER

A plastic strip is placed against the forehead to take a temperature reading. Some of these temperature strips may be left on the forehead to monitor the presence of a fever continually. These strips may display the temperature or change color to indicate a fever.

You can find a special infant pacifier thermometer that even changes color when the baby's temperature rises. Pharmacies, health and beauty stores, and supermarkets carry thermometers.

PULSE MEASUREMENT AND FITNESS TESTING

Electronics has made it possible to monitor several body functions at the same time with a unit that is no larger than a personal stereo. It measures heart rate in average beats, oxygen uptake, calories expended, and elapsed time. It is used to calculate target heart rates and can also calculate a fitness index based on age, sex, weight, and oxygen use.

This is one self-monitoring device that has more than one use, and may be especially important to someone with a cardiac condition. Ask your doctor or pharmacist about the availability of the newest entry in the pulse-monitoring field.

VISION TESTING

Most forms of vision testing can be performed in the home with eye charts akin to what you find in the doctor's office. You can screen yourself for visual acuity, astigmatism, color blindness, and macular degeneration. Many of the charts used for home vision testing are available at pharmacies and health and beauty stores, and through mail-order companies.

VISUAL ACUITY

The Snellen chart is what you see in doctors' offices. It has the large letters at the top and the smaller letters at the bottom. If you can read the ⅜ inch letters at 20 feet, your visual acuity is said to be 20/20.

ASTIGMATISM

This chart is somewhat like the face of a clock with all the numbers connected by diameter lines (12 to 6, 9 to 3, and so forth). The effect is a starburst, with all lines crossing in the center. When you look at the chart, all the lines should appear uniformly dark.

COLOR BLINDNESS

Home testing for color blindness is done using a multicolored chart in which a number has been hidden among the many colors. It is most often keyed to red and green or blue and yellow. A color-blind person would not be able to distinguish the number.

MACULAR DEGENERATION

The grid test (see page 78) is used to detect macular degeneration. The test consists of a grid with tiny squares and a dot at the center of the chart. Your ability to stare at the dot and see the smaller squares is very important. If any of the lines appear wavy or disappear, you should consult your eye-care professional.

EAR EXAMINATION

Young children often have more than their share of earaches and other ear problems. That's why parents can benefit from learning how to use the otoscope (a hand-held lighted instrument with a magnifying lens and a viewing cone) to monitor the health of the ear canal and the eardrum. Using an otoscope is not particularly difficult, and with a little effort you can become skilled at using it. You'll need some time and a willing patient.

The otoscope is a rather simple piece of equipment as medical equipment goes. You'll need to learn to identify the basic structure of the ear and eardrum, as well as the symptoms of ear infections. This includes identifying the normal color and shape of the eardrum, the location of the bones of the middle ear, and the signs of pressure behind the eardrum.

Otoscopes can be purchased at most pharmacies and through mail-order companies.

SELF-EXAM FOR DENTAL PLAQUE

Dental plaque is the unseen enemy of teeth and a major cause of tooth decay and gum disease. The best way to get rid of plaque is through proper daily brushing and flossing of the teeth. However, since it is virtually invisible, you need help in finding it. Enter the plaque disclosure tablet. Regular use of plaque-disclosing tablets will help you in your battle against tooth decay and gum disease.

This self-test is quick and easy to use. You need special disclosing tablets such as "Red-Kote" or "X-pose." After your regular brushing and flossing, chew one of the tablets and make sure you thoroughly mix it with your saliva. As the tablet dissolves, it leaves behind a red stain that adheres to the plaque.

You may need a small light and dental mirror to complete your examination. The darkest areas are those with the most plaque and other debris. Plaque-disclosing tablets and other dental self-care tools are available from dentists and pharmacies.

HOME BLOOD PRESSURE MONITORING

High blood pressure is often called a silent killer, because unlike other diseases it often remains hidden. You don't get a rash or sore spot, so you may have it but not know it. However, you can learn to monitor your own blood pressure.

You'll need a blood pressure cuff, or sphygmomanometer (sfig-mo-muh-nom-itur), as it is called, and a little practice. Blood pressure cuffs generally come in two varieties, manually operated cuffs and computerized cuffs. They both work the same way. It's just that the manual cuff requires a bit more work because you need to learn how to inflate the cuff, listen for the heartbeat, and read the blood pressure gauge. The computerized model does all the work for you.

Blood pressure home monitoring kits are available at most pharmacies and health and beauty stores, and through mail-order companies.

SELF-TESTING FOR LUNG FUNCTION

Self-tests for lung functions can be performed with or without special equipment. There are six generally recognized self-tests that you can perform at home.

MATCH TEST

Hold a lighted match about six inches from your mouth, take a deep breath, and then exhale as forcefully as you can, attempting to blow out the match. If you can perform this simple test without any problems, chances are you don't have any serious lung problems.

FORCED EXPIRATORY TEST

You'll need a stopwatch to count the seconds it takes to exhale all of your breath. Take a deep breath and, with your mouth open, exhale as fast as you can. The normal time is between two and six seconds. If it takes you longer than that, you may need additional testing.

You will need a peak flow meter (a device that measures the amount of air you exhale) and a spirometer (an instrument that measures the amount of air entering and leaving the lungs) for the following tests:

PEAK EXPIRATORY FLOW RATE

Take a deep breath and blow into the mouthpiece of the peak flow meter, which registers in liters the volume of air leaving your lungs. Repeat this test three times to establish a baseline. In subsequent tests any decrease from this baseline in the amount of air exhaled could indicate a potential problem and should be closely monitored.

FORCED VITAL CAPACITY AND FORCED EXPIRATORY VOLUME IN ONE SECOND

Use the spirometer for these tests. Take a deep breath and then blow into the mouthpiece of the spirometer as long and hard and fast as you can. This measures how much air you can expel from your lungs after a deep breath. Some spirometers will also calculate your Forced Expiratory Volume in One Second. This is a measure of how long it takes to expel at least 75 percent of your normal lung capacity in one second. If your measurement is less than 75 percent, it could indicate the need for further testing.

MAXIMUM VOLUNTARY VENTILATION

The purpose of this test is to measure the maximum volume of air that you can inhale and exhale in one minute. You'll need two things for this test: a spirometer and the Forced Vital Capacity reading from your earlier test. Hold the spirometer in your hand, and inhale and exhale as fast as you can for 15 seconds. Note the reading on the spirometer and multiply it by four. This gives you your MVV for one minute. You should repeat this process at least three times in order to determine your average MVV. The exact amount of air you are able to inhale and exhale is dependent on your age, body size, lung capacity, and general state of health. Your MVV should be about 15 to 20 times greater than your FVC reading. If your MVV falls short of this range, then it could indicate that you need to seek professional assistance for a complete pulmonary workup.

Peak flow monitors and spirometers may be purchased at pharmacies and through mail-order companies.

URINALYSIS

Simple-to-use home urinalysis products make it easy to monitor the workings of many body systems: the endocrine system, kidneys, liver, gallbladder, blood, spleen, bone marrow, and pancreas.

You'll need what are called dipsticks to perform the urinalysis. Dipsticks are specially treated papers that contain chemicals that react to the various components of urine. You can monitor the acidity (pH) and density (specific gravity) of urine, or you can check for blood, ketones (an indication of possible diabetes), and glucose.

Multiple-purpose dipsticks make it possible to perform a series of tests with one urine sample. There are also single-purpose dipsticks that monitor such things as glucose, vitamin C, and protein. Urine dipstick tests are available from pharmacies and through mail-order companies.

SELF-TESTING FOR URINARY TRACT INFECTIONS

Urinary tract infections (UTIs) are diseases that affect the kidneys, ureters, bladder, and urethra. When the urinary system has an infection, it can be downright painful and uncomfortable, and if left untreated, can lead to serious kidney disease. Self-tests for urinary tract infections can help identify the culprits causing the problem.

Three types of tests determine the presence of a urinary tract infection: cultures, leukocyte dipsticks, and nitrite dipsticks.

CULTURES

You place a sample of the urine on a specially prepared slide or tube. If a bacterium is present, it should grow in the medium.

LEUKOCYTE DIPSTICKS

This test checks the urine for the presence of white blood cells, which may indicate that an infection is present. An increase in white blood cells indicates that the body is fighting an infection.

NITRITE DIPSTICKS

This dipstick test looks for nitrites that are not normally present in the urine. A certain type of bacterium converts the nitrates in our diet to nitrites, and if nitrites are in the urine, then an infection may also be present.

Dipstick tests are available from pharmacies and through mail-order companies.

OVULATION AND PREGNANCY SELF-TEST

These two self-tests are listed together (but sold separately), because in a sense you can't have one without the other. Ovulation testing enables women to track their periods of maximum fertility and use that information to control their reproductive activities. Pregnancy testing enables women to confirm whether or not they are pregnant.

Ovulation testing is accomplished with a urine sample and a specially treated dipstick that detects the presence of a luteinizing hormone excreted during ovulation. (A luteinizing hormone is released by the pituitary gland, and in the female it stimulates the development of the corpus luteum, an increase which is a sign that the ovary has discharged its ovum.) The dipstick is placed in the urine and observed for any color change. Comparing the color to the guide supplied with the test kit will indicate whether or not the hormone is present.

Pregnancy testing is similar in that it also looks for a hormone that is produced only when a woman is pregnant. A urine sample is collected and mixed with a special reagent solution (a chemical that helps to identify the hormone). After it has been mixed, a special dipstick is used to test the solution. Changes in color indicate whether or not the woman is pregnant. Because there is always the chance of a mistake, it is advisable to repeat any pregnancy test.

Home tests for ovulation and pregnancy are available in most pharmacies, health and beauty stores, and even some supermarkets.

HOME BLOOD GLUCOSE MONITORING

Diabetics naturally have the most pressing need for blood glucose monitoring; however, even if you aren't diabetic, you may want to consider home blood glucose monitoring. This is especially true if there's any evidence of diabetes in your family. Home glucose monitoring enables diabetics to take control of their lives and take precautions against secondary illnesses such as kidney disease, blindness, nerve damage, and heart disease.

The glucose monitors of today are very sophisticated and quite accurate, a far cry from the early chemical dipsticks that many diabetics used. Two popular methods for monitoring glucose are reagent pads and glucose meters. The reagent pad changes color, depending on the amount of glucose in the blood, while the meter reads a strip of specially treated paper and produces a digital display.

A variety of equipment is available, from finger stick devices to glucose meters, and most of it can be found in the self-care section of pharmacies.

HOME THROAT CULTURES

Sore throats are generally associated with the cold and flu season and are caused by a virus. There is, however, another type of sore throat that is caused by a bacterium known as streptococcus, or strep for short. This type of sore throat, if not properly diagnosed and treated, can lead to other illnesses.

The only way to determine if a sore throat is caused by this bacterium is to take a throat specimen and culture it. If strep is present, it will grow in the culture.

Performing a throat culture test is a two-step process. Your physician can supply you with the specimen collection kit and show you how to collect the specimen. The collection kit is basically a large cotton swab that is carefully swept through the throat from side to side. Once you've collected the specimen, you return it to the physician or a laboratory.

The laboratory will grow the culture in a special oven and report the results to your physician. Because of the special equipment involved, you can't do the full test at home. However, by taking the specimen yourself, you save the cost of an extra visit to the doctor.

SELF-TEST FOR BREATH ALCOHOL

This type of test is very important if you're planning a night on the town and don't want to end up with a driving-while-intoxicated (DWI) citation on your driving record. Alcohol intoxication is fast becoming socially unacceptable, and there is much more emphasis on responsible drinking. Research has shown that alcohol enters the bloodstream very quickly, and before you know it, your blood alcohol level (BAC) is over the legal limit.

There are two basic types of monitors for checking your blood alcohol level: the balloon test and the electronic breath meter.

BALLOON TEST

The balloon test is probably the best known of the breath alcohol monitors. It consists of a balloon mouthpiece and a glass tube filled with specially treated crystals. As you blow into the balloon, your breath flows over the crystals, which change color according to the level of alcohol present.

ELECTRONIC BREATH METER

This type of monitor works on the same principle as the balloon test. As you blow through the mouthpiece of the meter, it automatically measures the amount of alcohol that is present. The display will signal whether or not your blood alcohol level is at or near the legal limit.

Breath alcohol monitors are available from pharmacies and through mail-order companies.

HOME SCREENING FOR BOWEL CANCER

Colorectal cancer is called the silent cancer, because people are reluctant to discuss it publicly. Yet it is responsible for some 60,000 cancer deaths each year. The home screening test for colorectal cancer is designed to detect the presence of hidden (occult) blood in the stool.

The advantage of using the home screening kit for colorectal cancer is that you can do it in the privacy of your home. In addition, when colorectal cancer is detected early, the chance of recovery is much better. There are three basic types of home screening: the stain method, the toilet paper test, and the pad test.

STAIN METHOD

A small stool specimen is collected and placed on a specially treated piece of paper. The presence of occult blood is determined after a staining solution is applied to the specimen. The stain will adhere to the occult blood.

TOILET PAPER TEST

Special toilet paper is used and then sprayed with a chemical disclosing agent. If occult blood is present, the paper will turn blue.

PAD TEST

This is probably the easiest test to use, since it only requires dropping a test pad in the toilet after a bowel movement. If occult blood is present, the pad will change color.

Home-screening tests for colorectal cancer are available from pharmacies and health and beauty stores, and through mail-order companies.

HOME TEST FOR PINWORMS

Pinworms usually infect children, but no one is immune from these intestinal parasites. The most commonly observed symptom is itching in the anal area, especially at night.

You don't need much more than a flashlight to conduct this test, since it's primarily one of observation. If you don't observe the worms, you may want to check for worm eggs, and for that you'll need a tape test.

It's best to check for pinworms at night when they are most active, and the threadlike adult worm can be observed. You simply shine the light over the anal area and note the presence or absence of worms. If there are no worms present, you may also want to check for worm eggs.

The pinworm egg test is done using a sticky tape. It is pressed over the anal area and collects the eggs. Because they are microscopic in size, you can't observe them with the naked eye, so in most cases you will have to take the tape to your doctor or a laboratory.

Medication to combat pinworms is available from pharmacies, or you can ask your doctor.

VAGINAL SELF-EXAM

The vaginal self-exam is intended to enable women to learn more about their bodies, and become better informed on the subject of gynecological health. Through routine examination and monitoring, they can learn how to spot indications of infections, irritations, or discharges. This information can then be used in conjunction with the professional care they are receiving.

You'll need the following equipment to perform a vaginal self-exam: a flashlight or other suitable light, a hand-held mirror, and a vaginal speculum (an instrument with two duck-bill blades that open to allow the viewing of the vaginal walls and cervix).

The examination is best done with your knees bent and the feet spread apart. The mirror should be placed in front of the vagina and should have a long handle so it's easy to reach. The speculum is then inserted into the vagina with the blades closed. After insertion, carefully turn the handle and open the blades. With the mirror positioned in front of the vagina, shine the light into the mirror, and reflect the light into the vagina.

It's a good idea to use the self-exam information that's included with the speculum kit, since this describes the normal appearance of the vagina and cervix. Any irregularities should be noted and mentioned to your health-care professional.

Vaginal self-exam kits are available from pharmacies and women's health centers, and through mail-order companies.

BREAST SELF-EXAM

See self-exam on pages 87–89.

TESTICULAR SELF-EXAM

See self-exam on pages 91–92.

SELF-TEST FOR ERECTION PROBLEMS

The test most often used to detect erection problems is the Nocturnal Penile Tumescence Stamp Test, or NPT. Impotence, the inability to achieve an erection, may be caused by physical or psychological factors, or a combination of both.

The NPT test can help determine whether or not a man's ability to achieve an erection is physical or psychological. It is considered normal for a man to have one to four erections during periods of deep sleep known as REM (rapid eye movement) sleep. This information led to the development of the stamp test.

This test is relatively easy to perform, and the only thing you need is a roll of stamps. You may use postage stamps or you can order a roll of specially designed stamps for this purpose. You will need a strip of four to six stamps and a total of twelve to eighteen stamps for the three-night test.

You select the first strip of stamps and place them around the penis before going to bed. Upon awakening, examine the stamps to determine if they are broken or if there are any perforations between stamps. If the stamps are broken or perforated in any way, it probably means that you had an erection sometime during your sleep. In any event, it's recommended that you repeat the test for three consecutive nights.

Additional information on the stamp test and tests for impotence can be obtained from any trained sexual counselor. Ask your pharmacist for information on the availability of stamps for the NPT test.

SINUS TRANSILLUMINATION

At one time or another, nearly everyone has experienced some sort of sinus problem. The all-too-familiar pain around the eyes, the stuffy nose, and the ever-present headache are all reminders of the discomfort brought on by sinus problems.

You can save yourself some time and money if you learn how to conduct an examination of your own sinuses using a flashlight. Both the maxillary (the sinuses below your eyes and on either side of your face) and frontal (those above your eyes) can be examined. This type of examination is known as transillumination, a fancy way of saying that you're going to shine a light through your sinuses.

In addition to the flashlight, you'll need a darkened room and a mirror. Once in the room, stand in front of the mirror, open your mouth, and carefully insert the flashlight. Make sure that you keep your mouth closed so no light can escape. With all that light in your mouth it should be easy to see your maxillary sinuses. Clear sinuses will appear bright, while congested sinuses will be cloudy.

Examine your frontal sinuses by placing the light just under the bony ridge above your eyes. You may find a penlight is better suited for examining the frontal sinuses. Once again, compare the amount of light that is visible from each sinus to determine whether it is clear or congested.

SELF-TEST FOR BODY FAT COMPOSITION

You don't need to be an Olympic athlete to be interested in your body fat composition. Researchers who study fitness have developed some general guidelines on the subject of percentages of fat to body weight.

Using the standard of 19 percent body fat for men and 22 percent for women, you can test yourself to determine how well you measure up to these standards. The researchers also note that the percentage of body fat for athletically inclined men and women should be 15 and 18 percent, respectively.

The easiest form of body fat testing you can do is the skinfold thickness test. You'll need a special caliper to measure the thickness of the skinfolds taken on various parts of the body. The best location to do a skinfold test is the forearm or the area below the shoulder blade. You pinch the skin and pull it away from the body until you have a fold of skin that can be measured with the caliper. Place the caliper over the fold and slowly close it. When you can't close it any farther, take the reading from the scale on the caliper. Record this reading on the chart supplied with the caliper kit.

Use the body fat tables that come with the caliper to make a determination of your percentage of body fat. Body fat composition kits are available from pharmacies and through mail-order companies. You might even check with fitness clubs in your area.

For further information on these and other self-tests, two excellent sources are *Do-It-Yourself Medical Testing* and *The People's Book of Medical Tests*.

BIBLIOGRAPHY

Basic Books

Children's Friendships, by Zick Rubin. Cambridge, Mass.: Harvard University Press, 1980.

Counseling in the Elementary and Middle Schools, by James J. Muro and Don C. Dinkmeyer. Dubuque, Iowa: William C. Brown, 1977.

Do-It-Yourself Medical Testing (3rd ed.), by Cathey Pinckney and Edward Pinckney. New York: Facts on File, 1983.

A Good Enough Parent, by Dr. Bruno Bettelheim. New York: Knopf, 1987.

X rays: Health Effects of Common Exams, by John W. Gofman, M.D., and Egan O'Connor. San Francisco: Sierra Club Books, 1985.

Health Shock, by Martin Weitz. Englewood Cliffs, N.J.: Prentice-Hall, 1982.

A Healthy State, by Victor W. Sidel and Ruth Sidel. New York: Pantheon, 1983.

Helping Your Children Cope with Stress, by Avis Brenner, Ed.D. Lexington, Mass.: Lexington Books, 1984.

The Malpractitioners, by John Guinther. New York: Doubleday, 1978.

Medication Errors: Causes and Prevention, by Neil M. Davis and Michael R. Cohen. Philadelphia: George F. Stickley, 1981.

Mind and Media, by Patricia Marks Greenfield. Cambridge, Mass.: Harvard University Press, 1984.

A Parent's Guide to Childhood Symptoms, by Richard Martin, M.D. New York: St. Martin's Press, 1982.

Parents' Guide to Raising a Gifted Child, by Dr. Bruno Bettelheim. Boston: Little, Brown, 1985.

The People's Book of Medical Tests, by Tom Ferguson, M.D., and David Sobel, M.D. New York: Summit Books, 1985.

The Rights of Patients: The Basic ACLU Guide to Patient Rights, by George J. Annas. Carbondale: Southern Illinois University Press, 1989.

The Rights of the Critically Ill, by John A. Robertson. New York: Bantam Books, 1983.

When to Say No to Surgery, by Robert G. Schneider, M.D. Englewood Cliffs, N.J.: Prentice-Hall, 1982.

More Books to Help You Maximize Your Health and Fitness

Advanced First Aid and Emergency Care, by the American Red Cross. New York: Doubleday, 1986.

Advice for the Patient: Drug Information in Lay Language (9th ed.). Rockville, Md.: United States Pharmacopeial Convention, 1989.

Alternative Medicine: A Guide to Natural Therapies, by Andrew Stanway. New York: Penguin, 1982.

The American Medical Association Family Medical Guide (rev. ed.), edited by Jeffery R. Kuntz, M.D., and Asher J. Finkel, M.D. New York: Random House, 1987.

The American Medical Association Home Medical Adviser, edited by Charles Clayman, M.D., et al. New York: Random House, 1988.

Anatomy of an Illness as Perceived by the Patient, by Norman Cousins. New York: Norton, 1979.

Cecil Textbook of Medicine (17th ed.), edited by James Wyngaarden and Lloyd Smith. Philadelphia: W. B. Saunders, 1985.

The Columbia University College of Physicians and Surgeons Complete Home Medical Guide (revised ed.), edited by Donald F. Tapley, M.D., et al. New York: Crown, 1989.

Complete Book of Vitamins and Minerals for Health, by the editors of *Prevention* magazine. Emmaus, Pa.: Rodale Press, 1988.

Complete Guide to Healing Your Body Naturally, by Gary Null. New York: McGraw-Hill, 1988.

Consumerism in Medicine: Challenging Physician Authority, by Marie Haug and Bebe Lavin. Beverly Hills, Calif.: Sage Publications, 1983.

Current Medical Diagnosis and Treatment (26th ed.), by Marcus Krupp and Milton L. Chatton. Los Altos, Calif.: Appleton-Lange, 1987.

Current Surgical Diagnosis and Treatment (7th ed.), by L. W. Way. Los Altos, Calif.: Appleton-Lange, 1985.

Dorland's Illustrated Medical Dictionary (26th ed.). Philadelphia: W. B. Saunders, 1985.

Drug Information for the Consumer. Mount Vernon, N.Y.: Consumer Reports Books, 1987.

The Essential Guide to Prescription Drugs (6th ed.), by James W. Long. New York: Harper & Row, 1988.

Fighting Disease, by Ellen Michaud and Alice Feinstein. Emmaus, Pa.: Rodale Press, 1989.

The Food and Drug Interaction Books, by Brian L. Morgan. New York: Simon & Schuster, 1986.

General Ophthalmology (11th ed.), by Daniel Vaughn and Taylor Asbury. Los Altos, Calif.: Appleton-Lange, 1986.

Harrison's Principles of Internal Medicine (11th ed.), edited by Eugene Braunwald, M.D., et al. New York: McGraw-Hill, 1987.

The Healing Heart, by Norman Cousins. New York: Avon Books, 1984.

Health Care U.S.A.: Where to Find the Best Answers to Your Family Medical Health Problems, by Jean Carper. New York: Prentice-Hall, 1987.

The Home Medical Handbook, by Jack I. Stern, M.D., and David L. Carroll. New York: Morrow, 1987.

How to Evaluate and Select a Nursing Home, by R. Barker Bausell, Michael A. Rooney, and Charles B. Inlander. Reading, Mass.: Addison-Wesley, 1988.

How to Keep Your Child Fit from Birth to Six, by Bonnie Prudden. New York: Ballantine Books, 1986.

Mastering Pain: A Twelve-Step Program for Coping with Chronic Pain, by Richard A. Sternbach. New York: Putnam, 1987.

Mayo Clinic Diet Manual: A Handbook of Dietary Practices (5th ed.). Philadelphia: W. B. Saunders, 1981.

Medical Self-Care Book of Women's Health, by Sadja Greenwood and Michael Castleman. Garden City, N.Y.: Doubleday, 1987.

Medicare Made Easy, by Charles B. Inlander and Charles K. MacKay. Reading, Mass.: Addison-Wesley, 1989.

Medicine on Trial, by Charles B. Inlander, Lowell Levin, and Ed Weiner. New York: Prentice-Hall, 1988.

The New Good Housekeeping Family Health and Medical Guide. New York: Hearst Books, 1989.

The New Our Bodies, Ourselves, by the Boston Women's Health Book Collective. New York: Simon & Schuster, 1984.

The New People's Pharmacy Book: A Guide to Prescription Drugs, by Joe Graedon. New York: Bantam Books, 1985.

Over the Counter Pills That Don't Work, by Joel Kaufman et al. Washington, D.C.: Public Citizen Health Research Group, 1983.

Patient Beware, by Cynthia Carver. Scarborough, Ontario: Prentice-Hall, 1984.

The Patient's Guide to Medical Tests (3rd ed., revised and enlarged), by Cathey Pinckney and Edward Pinckney. New York: Facts on File, 1987.

Peace, Love and Healing, by Bernie S. Siegel, M.D. New York: Harper & Row, 1989.

The People's Medical Manual, by Howard R. Lewis and Martha E. Lewis. Garden City, N.Y.: Doubleday, 1986.

The Pharmacist's Prescription: Your Complete Guide to Over-the-Counter Remedies, by F. James Grogan. Riverside, N.J.: Rawson Associates, 1987.

Rodale's Encyclopedia of Natural Home Remedies, by Mark Bricklin. Emmaus, Pa.: Rodale Press, 1982.

Standard First Aid and Personal Safety, by the American Red Cross. Garden City, N.Y.: Doubleday, 1986.

Staying Healthy Without Medicine, by Daniel P. Marshall, J. Gregory Rabold, and Edgar S. Wilson. Chicago: Nelson Hall, 1983.

Take Care of Yourself: A Consumer's Guide to Medical Care (3rd ed.), by Donald M. Vickery, M.D., and James F. Fries, M.D. Reading, Mass.: Addison-Wesley, 1986.

Take This Book to the Hospital with You (rev. ed.), by Charles B. Inlander and Ed Weiner. New York: Pantheon, 1991.

Third Opinion, by John M. Fink. Garden City, N.Y.: Avery Publishing Group, 1988.

When to Say No to Surgery, by Robert G. Schneider, M.D. Englewood Cliffs, N.J.: Prentice-Hall, 1982.

Womancare: A Gynecological Guide to Your Body, by Linda Madras and Jane Patterson. New York: Avon, 1984.

Worst Pills, Best Pills, by Sidney Wolfe, M.D., et al. Washington, D.C.: Public Citizen Health Research Group, 1988.

Your Medical Rights, by Charles B. Inlander and Eugene Pavalon. Boston: Little, Brown, 1990.

ACKNOWLEDGMENTS

"Test Your Overall Nutrition Knowledge" originally titled "Eating Well: Here's a Quiz to Test Your Overall Nutrition Knowledge" by Marian Burros, *The New York Times*. Copyright © 1989 by The New York Times Company. Reprinted by permission.

"Are You Up On Your Facts About Fat?" by Ken Levine, originally in *Reader's Digest*. Copyright 1989 Ken Levine. Reprinted with permission.

Chart for "Are You at Risk of Obesity?" reprinted with permission of Steven B. Heymsfield, M.D.

"Test Yourself: Vitamins," *Better Nutrition for Today's Living*, June 1990, reprinted with permission.

"Do You Know Where the Sodium is in Your Diet?" reprinted from *Blood Pressure: Questions You Have . . . Answers You Need*, People's Medical Society, 1984.

"Test Your Health IQ," reprinted by permission of *Executive.Edge*. Copyright 1990 Rodale Press, Inc. All rights reserved.

"How Fit Are You?" by Carol Krucoff, originally in *The Washington Post*. Reprinted with permission of the author.

"A Quick Test for Macular Disease: Thief of Central Vision" by Richard L. Pharo. Reprinted with the permission of Citizens for Eye Research, a national nonprofit public education agency working to prevent blindness.

Test for "Glaucoma: Are You at Risk?" from "Take This Test and Save Your Sight" by George L. Spaeth, M.D. Used with permission.

"How's Your Hearing?" reprinted with permission from American Academy of Otolaryngology—Head and Neck Surgery, Alexandria, Va.

Two tables for "Do Your Height and Weight See Eye to Eye?" courtesy *Statistical Bulletin*, Metropolitan Life Insurance Company.

Material in "How to Determine Your Target Heart Rate" from *The Aerobics Program for Total Well-Being* by Kenneth H. Cooper, M.D., M.P.H., copyright © 1982 by Kenneth H. Cooper. Used with permission of Bantam Books, a division of Bantam, Doubleday, Dell Publishing Group, Inc.

"How to do Breast Self-Examination," by permission of the American Cancer Society.

"Health IQ Test: Osteoporosis," reprinted with permission of *Lake Echoes Health News*, Our Lady of the Lake Regional Medical Center, Baton Rouge, LA.

"Vasectomy Myths: How Many Have You Fallen For?" reprinted by permission of *Men's Health Newsletter.* Copyright 1989 Rodale Press, Inc. All rights reserved.

"The Rockport Fitness Walking Test" reprinted by permission of The Rockport Company from "The Rockport Guide to Fitness Walking." © 1989 The Rockport Company. All rights reserved.

"What's Your Parenting Quotient?" reprinted by permission of *Rodale's Children Magazine.* Copyright 1988 Rodale Press, Inc. All rights reserved.

"How Balanced is Your Child's Diet?" reprinted by permission of *Rodale's Children Magazine.* Copyright 1988 Rodale Press, Inc. All rights reserved.

"Is Your Child Allergic?" reprinted by permission of *Rodale's Children Magazine.* Copyright 1986 Rodale Press, Inc. All rights reserved.

Test for "Is My Baby's Hearing Normal?" reprinted with permission from American Academy of Otolaryngology—Head and Neck Surgery, Inc., Alexandria, VA.

"Simple Do-It-Yourself Scoliosis Check," reprinted by permission of *Rodale's Children Magazine.* Copyright 1986 Rodale Press, Inc. All rights reserved.

"How Fit Are Your Kids?" reprinted by permission of *Rodale's Children Magazine.* Copyright 1986 Rodale Press, Inc. All rights reserved.

"Is Your Playground Safe?" reprinted by permission of *Rodale's Children Magazine.* Copyright 1988 Rodale Press, Inc. All rights reserved.

"How to Choose the Right Pediatrician," reprinted by permission of *Rodale's Children Magazine.* Copyright 1987 Rodale Press, Inc. All rights reserved.

"Parent's Rights: Do You Know Where You Stand?" reprinted from *Your Child's Health,* People's Medical Society, 1986.

"A Test About Unnecessary Testing," *People's Medical Society Newsletter,* October 1990.

"Does Your Doctor Treat You with the Respect You Deserve?" reprinted from the People's Medical Society, "Code of Practice."

FOR THE BEST IN PAPERBACKS, LOOK FOR THE

In every corner of the world, on every subject under the sun, Penguin represents quality and variety—the very best in publishing today.

For complete information about books available from Penguin—including Pelicans, Puffins, Peregrines, and Penguin Classics—and how to order them, write to us at the appropriate address below. Please note that for copyright reasons the selection of books varies from country to country.

In the United Kingdom: For a complete list of books available from Penguin in the U.K., please write to *Dept E.P., Penguin Books Ltd, Harmondsworth, Middlesex, UB7 0DA.*

In the United States: For a complete list of books available from Penguin in the U.S., please write to *Dept BA, Penguin*, Box 120, Bergenfield, New Jersey 07621-0120.

In Canada: For a complete list of books available from Penguin in Canada, please write to *Penguin Books Ltd, 2801 John Street, Markham, Ontario L3R 1B4.*

In Australia: For a complete list of books available from Penguin in Australia, please write to the *Marketing Department, Penguin Books Ltd, P.O. Box 257, Ringwood, Victoria 3134.*

In New Zealand: For a complete list of books available from Penguin in New Zealand, please write to the *Marketing Department, Penguin Books (NZ) Ltd, Private Bag, Takapuna, Auckland 9.*

In India: For a complete list of books available from Penguin, please write to *Penguin Overseas Ltd, 706 Eros Apartments, 56 Nehru Place, New Delhi, 110019.*

In Holland: For a complete list of books available from Penguin in Holland, please write to *Penguin Books Nederland B.V., Postbus 195, NL-1380AD Weesp, Netherlands.*

In Germany: For a complete list of books available from Penguin, please write to *Penguin Books Ltd, Friedrichstrasse 10-12, D-6000 Frankfurt Main 1, Federal Republic of Germany.*

In Spain: For a complete list of books available from Penguin in Spain, please write to *Longman, Penguin España, Calle San Nicolas 15, E-28013 Madrid, Spain.*

In Japan: For a complete list of books available from Penguin in Japan, please write to *Longman Penguin Japan Co Ltd, Yamaguchi Building, 2-12-9 Kanda Jimbocho, Chiyoda-Ku, Tokyo 101, Japan.*